MW00639533

LED and Light Therapy: CLINICAL PROCEDURES

First Edition

By Curtis Turchin, MA, DC

Disclaimer

It is the responsibility of the practitioner to gain the knowledge of and comply with federal, state, and local laws regarding the use of light and lasers for the treatment of any condition. The content and information in this book is educational only and is designed as an addendum to formal training in light and laser therapy. It is not a complete course and should not be relied upon for the purpose of treating an individual.

This book is not a substitute for professional medical advice, care, diagnosis or treatment. The treatment of any disease or syndrome should be under the auspices of a qualified physician or therapist.

Dr. Curtis Turchin does not warrant or assume any legal liability or responsibility for the accuracy, completeness, or usefulness of any information, apparatus, product or process disclosed in his book, seminars, or other educational activities. Therefore, Dr. Curtis Turchin is not liable for any kind of loss, risk, or other problem, which is sustained as a result of consulting this book or from using information obtained in any of his books or seminars.

Contact Information

Websites: www.CurtisTurchin.com
www.GentleMobilization.com
Phone: Dr. Turchin 707-206-7272

ISBN-13: 9781947962033

Printed in the United States

Introduction: Using This Book

This is a clinical text to help you effectively use light therapy in your clinic. It is designed for almost any type of LED or light therapy product.

Order of Book

The treatment chapters are divided into anatomical regions of the body. The areas are Head and Face, Spine and Pelvis, Upper Extremity, Lower Extremity, Brain, and Systemic conditions. Within each anatomical region, the conditions are in alphabetic order. All diagrams are grouped at the end of each anatomical region so that you can refer to either the text or the diagram, depending on your clinical need.

SOAP Notes

Healthcare demands that practitioners document their findings. For that reason, each condition is organized by the SOAP format. This refers to the Subjective Symptoms, Objective Findings, Assessment, and treatment Plan. This has been designed to help you understand the condition and aid in organizing your assessment and treatment of the patient. There are two "P's." One Plan is your light treatment Plan and the other is your adjunctive treatment Plan. Because there are a wide variety of modalities available, only the most commonly used adjunctive treatment techniques are included.

Diagrams

In the diagrams, the stationary application of light to a single point on the skin is represented by dots and arrows. Smaller LED devices can apply light to a discrete point. For ease of use, the diagrams are only front and back views of the body. Therefore, any point that is applied to the side of the body not pictured is noted by an arrow and the frontal, visible view of the skin is demonstrated by a dot. These points correspond to anatomical locations, not acupuncture points.

Shading denotes that the light is applied in smooth, even strokes called Painting, which is like a slower, more methodical ultrasound application. This is described in the first chapter, Science of Light Therapy. Most conditions respond to both Point and Painting techniques.

Recommended Dosages

The recommended dosages in this text are based on using an LED with a total output power of between 10 and 10,000 mW. Please refer to the chart at the beginning of each DIAGRAM section for details on dosages for any device between 10 and 10,000 mW.

Ice and Heat

When the application of ice or heat is recommended, it is assumed that the patient can, depending on the practitioner's bias, use ice in the most acute stage, progress to alternating ice and heat as they become subacute, and use heat when the condition is not characterized by serious inflammation.

Suggestions

Light therapy is a new science compared to other modalities used in rehabilitation. Thus, our understanding is changing quickly. If you have information that you feel should be included in this book, or you find something inconsistent with research or your experience, please feel free to email the author. His email address is CurtisTurchin@gmail.com.

Contents

Science of Light Therapy

Overview of Light and Laser Therapy

This book has been designed as a handbook for the clinical use of LED therapy. Although it includes a short overview of physics, physiology, and the history of light, these subjects have been purposely limited to maintain the focus on the clinical aspects of laser therapy.

History

The ancient Greeks, Romans, and Egyptians used light therapy and applied heat to tender points in the human body to relieve symptoms of many syndromes.

In 1903, Nils Finsen, a Danish medical doctor, was given the Nobel Prize for successfully treating tuberculosis, rickets and lupus vulgaris with ultraviolet light. This was the first recognized application of artificial light to cure disease.

In 1923, the Russian researcher Alexander Gurwitsch first detected that cells emit infrared light as a means of intercellular communication. He observed that this light could be transmitted from a test tube to another adjacent one without any physical contact between them. He termed this infrared emission "mitogenetic radiation."

In 1967, Dr. Endre Mester, a professor of surgery in Hungary, performed a revolutionary series of experiments that first documented the healing effect of lasers. In his earliest study he discovered that tissue growth was accelerated with laser therapy. His later experiments documented not only improved healing with light therapy, but also demonstrated that the healing was a systemic and not a local phenomenon. His work stimulated many other researchers in Europe and Eastern Europe to appreciate the value of laser therapy, long before it was appreciated in Asia, Africa, and the Americas.

By the 1970s, light and laser therapy was beginning to attract attention in Eastern Europe, China, and the Soviet Union; thus, much of the early research emanates from these regions. Over the following ten years, light and laser therapy spread to Western Europe and quickly became popular as a physical therapy modality. However, many of the lasers used during this period produced only 5 to 50 mW of power and lacked the effectiveness of modern, more powerful lasers.

There has been a recent surge in the use of light therapy all over the world, particularly in surgery, dentistry, and physical therapy. In the area of physical therapy, light is being used by physical and occupational therapists, chiropractors, osteopaths, and acupuncturists because of its ability to relieve pain, stimulate healing, and create a wide variety of beneficial systemic effects.

Lasers and LEDs

In the area of physical therapy two types of light sources are used. They are Laser Diodes (LD) and Light Emitting Diodes (LED). Usually they are visible red (VR) or infrared (IR). Most of the popular diodes emit light in the 600–900 nanometer wavelength range. Lasers are monochromatic, thus emitting a single color of light. To the naked eye, LEDs also emit a single color; however, they actually emit over a narrow wavelength range of about 30 nm.

LEDs vs. Bright Light Therapy

In this book we are going to focus on using LEDs for many types of therapy. However, when we use the term "Light Therapy" we are not talking about "Bright Light Therapy." Bright Light Therapy is a way to treat seasonal affective disorder (SAD) and certain other conditions by exposure to artificial light. SAD is a type of depression that occurs usually in the fall or winter and is more common in northern latitudes. Bright Light Therapy is used as a substitute for sunlight and has been shown to reduce the depressive effects from increased darkness during the winter months.

LEDs vs. Lasers

For many years, clinicians have used laser therapy for healing all types of injuries including sprains and strains, postoperative care, wound care, pain relief, and inflammation control. More recently, light-emitting diodes (LEDs) have become popular for many of the same applications because studies show that, for most applications, they are as effective and much less expensive than lasers.

Because the world is steadily using more LEDs for home lighting, automotive use, and in many types of health care and computer applications, the cost of LED diodes has dropped dramatically and the quality and power of LEDs has increased much faster than with laser diodes.

Laser diodes have both similarities and differences to LEDs in terms of construction. Both are produced from similar "sandwiches" of semiconductor materials to produce light.

There are differences between laser and LED light therapy, and each has its strengths and weaknesses. In general, if you want a lot of power in a small space or for surgery, you would choose to use a laser. However, when treating larger areas, LEDs are safer and much less expensive.

LASER, which stands for Light Amplification by Stimulated Emission of Radiation, is created when electrons become energized from an electrical current. They are then emitted as energized photons in a relatively narrow beam called coherent light.

In contrast, LEDs emit light in a broader range. This more divergent beam makes them potentially less harmful to the eyes and other sensitive areas. Still, they exert a similar effect on tissues as lasers.

A leading scientist in the area of light therapy, Dr. Tina Karu, says, "No significant difference was found for growth stimulation regardless of whether the light used was generated by a laser or from light of the same wavelength from a filtered incandescent lamp."

In a NASA-sponsored study published in 2001, scientists found LED therapy to be effective for fast wound healing and pain reduction.

There are a number of opinions about which is better and there are clinicians who prefer one or the other.

Kendric Smith, a retired Professor Emeritus of Stanford University, said in 2005 that "all too often the laser phototherapy literature is written as if a laser is magical. Laser radiation follows (except for coherence) all of the same laws of physics and chemistry that the same wavelength of radiation from a conventional (non-coherent or LED) light source follows."

Other more recent studies demonstrate the feasibility of using a LED lamp as alternative to laser source. The main characteristic is not the light coherence but achieving a certain concentration of light of the appropriate wavelength. Researchers have concluded that the efficacy was achieved satisfactorily by LEDs and had the added benefits of convenience, accessibility, and safety.

How to Choose an LED Device

1. The first thing to consider is whether you want to place the device on the spot you want to treat or whether you want LEDs embedded in fabric that you can strap on your body.

   a. Strap-on devices sound easier, but they take a long time to produce results because they are very low power. There are many complaints in front of the FDA due to burns from strap-on LEDs. Usual treatment times for one area are about 20–30 minutes.

   b. Handheld LEDs are great if they are powerful. Look for one with 5,000 milliwatts or higher. The higher the power the faster the results. Usual treatment times are 1–2 minutes for one area.

2. Lower power LEDs take a long time to treat any significant injury. Look for an LED with 5,000–10,000 milliwatts as treatment times are very fast: usually 1–2 minutes per area. You can find devices like this through physical therapy and chiropractic dealers, Amazon, and other online stores.

Lasers Are Coherent, LEDs Are Not

The photons emanating from a laser are highly organized, directional, and termed "coherent light." Note in the picture below how the laser light is coherent, or "in-phase" and the LED light is non-coherent or "out of phase."

Notice how the laser light waves are "in-phase"

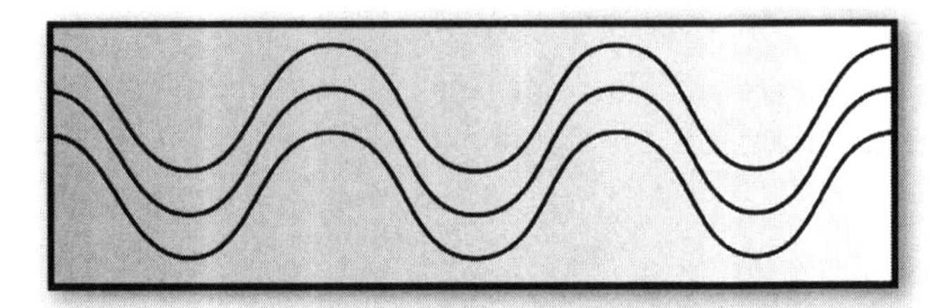

Notice how the LED light waves are "out of phase"

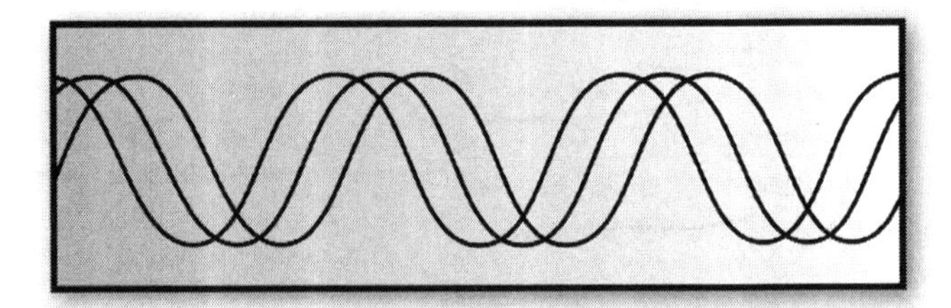

How Do We Measure Wavelength?

Light travels in a wave as depicted in the diagram below. We can characterize the light by its wavelength, which is the distance between successive peaks (or valleys) in the wave. We measure the wavelength of light in nanometers (nm).

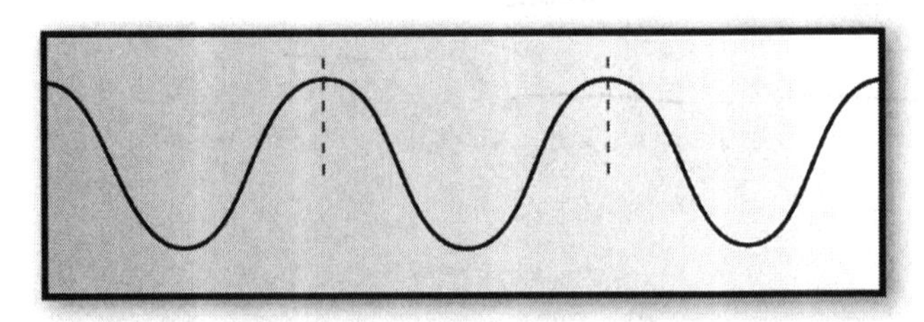

The length of 1 nanometer is 1 billionth of a meter. One thousand nm's equals one micron, which is a millionth of a meter. Thus, a 940 nm laser has a wavelength that is almost one micron. By comparison, the size of this dot (.), used as a period, is about 400 microns or 1/64 inch.

Electromagnetic Spectrum

The diagram on the next page shows the range of emissions called the electromagnetic spectrum. Note that the more damaging emissions, such as x-rays and ultraviolet light, are the shorter wavelengths. The extreme power of these short wavelengths can break the bonds of atoms and produce ions, and for that reason these shorter wavelengths are sometimes called ionizing radiation. Typically, at the other end of the spectrum, radiation in the infrared or visible red spectrum does not cause ionization, but it does generate heat when absorbed in tissue.

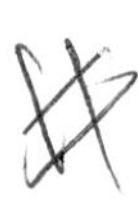

Water has very high absorption for light in wavelengths longer than 1500 nm, and since water is the major constituent of muscle tissue, this radiation does not penetrate significantly below the skin. We thus are left with an optimum treatment window which is the optical window, between approximately 600 nm to 900 nm where the radiation does not cause ionization and can penetrate beneath the skin to affect the underlying tissue. This is well visualized in the chart below. In the field of LED therapy, we use the term optical window to describe the range of 600–900 nm, because LEDs that have a wavelength greater than 900 nm produce a lot of heat and are more uncomfortable than the LEDs of shorter wavelengths with the same output power.

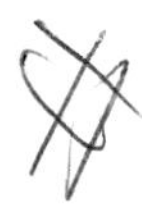

Note in the diagram below that light in the 600–900 nm wavelength is in the "optical window." This range of wavelengths is most likely to penetrate deeply into the tissues because the photons are not strongly absorbed by hemoglobin or water. When light is absorbed by hemoglobin and water it will be absorbed in the circulatory system and prevented from deeper penetration.

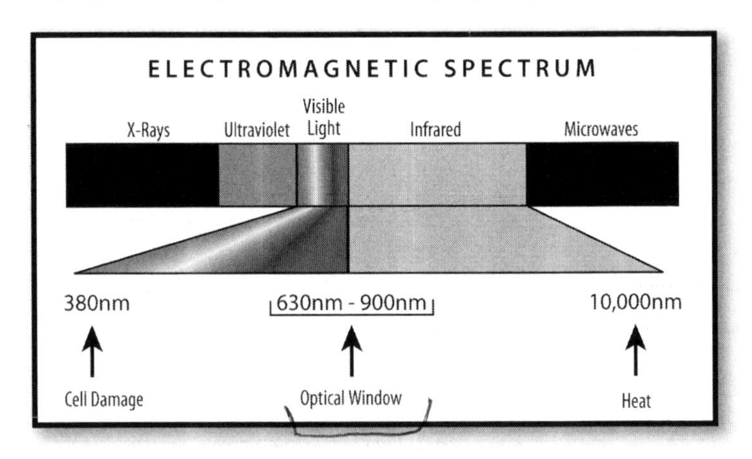

Depth of Light Penetration

The accepted depth of penetration of an LED depends on its wavelength, but, on average, penetrates about 5–7 cm (2–3+ in.). The majority of photons are absorbed in the first few millimeters. As the beam passes into the body, more superficial tissues absorb most of the photons, thus reducing the number of photons that reach deeper layers. However, as these photons enter the body, they create a powerful physiological effect by inducing local metabolic changes and the creation of second messengers. Second messengers are molecules that relay signals received at receptors on the cell surface that target molecules in the nucleus of the cell to modify physiological and genetic information.

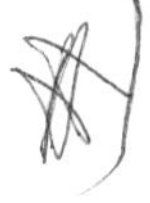

Second messengers also serve to greatly amplify the strength of the signal, causing massive changes in the biochemical activities within the cell. Thus, as the effect of the photons diminishes with increasing depth, the physiological effects rapidly multiply, creating a profound and systemic effect. This is how photons quickly create systemic effects. It was Mester's experiments in 1966–67 that first documented the widespread, systemic effect of light therapy.

In general, it is well accepted that longer wavelengths, such as 800–900 nm, penetrate slightly deeper than shorter wavelengths, such as 600–700 nm. However, these differences are small and can be overcome by power. Thus, it is most important, when choosing an LED device, to balance wavelength and power.

Generally, lasers are more deeply penetrating, but LEDs are less expensive, slightly more superficial, and are very effective when used in unattended LED pads or large laser clusters. Assuming a similar wavelength, a more powerful LED will provide faster results.

Important Terms and Parameters

3. Treatment time is expressed in seconds (sec). This is the most important parameter because it determines total dose.
4. Power is expressed in milliwatts (mW) or Watts (W). 1,000 mW is one Watt. The terms 1,000 milliwatts and 1 Watt are interchangeable.
5. Total dose or energy is expressed in joules (J). This is the power multiplied by the time, Watts x seconds.
6. Wavelength is expressed in nanometers (nm).
7. The projection or intensity of an LED is measured in millicandelas (mcd).

Light Energy Expressed in Joules

Light energy is expressed in joules (J). This energy is the result of multiplying the number of watts by the treatment time expressed in seconds.

Energy (joules) = Power (Watts) x Time (Seconds)

Some scientists describe a joule as a "Watt-Second," signifying that the number of watts multiplied by the number of seconds is the output in joules. Therefore:

1. A 2,000 mW LED (2 Watt) applied for 60 seconds, delivers 120 joules of energy.
    a. 2 W x 60 secs = 120 joules
2. A 1,000 mW LED (1 Watt) applied for 60 seconds, delivers 60 joules of energy.
    a. 1 W x 60 secs = 60 joules
3. A 500 mW (.5W) LED would deliver 30 joules of energy in 60 seconds.
    a. 0.5W x 60 secs = 30 joules
4. A 250 mW (.25W) LED would produce 15 joules of energy in 60 seconds
    a. 0.25W x 60 secs = 15 joules

How Much Light is Absorbed?

It is important that light be applied to clean skin, free from extra oils or creams. Oil will reduce the penetration of the photons by reflecting them off of the skin surface. We have an acronym for how the penetration of photons can occur: "R.A.T.S.," which stands for Reflection, Absorption, Transmission, and Scattering.

As you can see in the diagram below, light will react in varied ways with different types of surfaces and materials. For example, light will reflect off of any oily surface, will be absorbed and transmitted through many cells and will scatter off of metal and plastic implants.

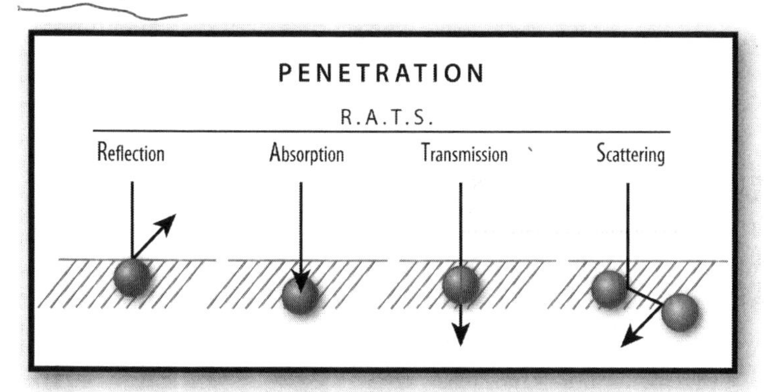

Skin Contact

Ideally, the LED should be applied directly on the skin. If the structure you are treating is buried deep beneath adipose tissue, pressure should be applied to the device to increase the depth of contact and move the beam closer to the area being treated. This also displaces fluids, such as blood, preventing too many of the photons from being absorbed on their way to the desired tissue. However, when treating wounds to prevent contamination, keep the probe about 1/4 to 1/2 inch above the skin.

SOAP Notes

If you are a professional, good note taking is important in any medical treatment. Always note the Subjective, Objective, Assessment, and Planning information in your daily notes.

Subjective stands for the patient's symptoms, Objective describes any objective observations and/or orthopedic testing, Assessment is the patient's diagnosis or response to treatment, and Plan refers to your treatment plan or what therapy was provided. In the treatment Plan you can note the following factors:

1. NECESSARY: Treatment time in seconds. This is the most important parameter to note as it determines the total dose, since typically the probe power is fixed.
2. NECESSARY: The anatomical location treated.
3. NECESSARY: Total output power of your device in mW or W. If you only use one probe, this would be optional since you only have one laser instrument.
4. NECESSARY: Wavelength of your device. If you only use one device, this would again be optional.
5. OPTIONAL: The total dose or energy in joules. This can be calculated based on treatment time.

Titration is important because, based on the above principles, providing too much light will inhibit the potential healing effects of light therapy.

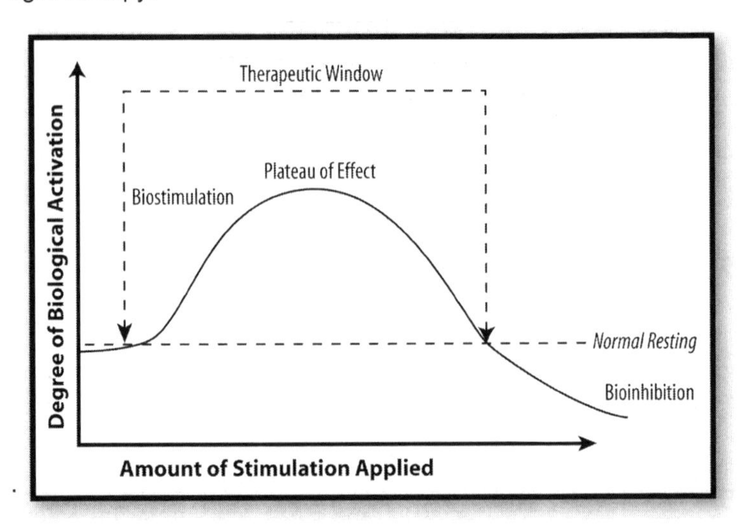

LED Safety

There are still a number of safety precautions to consider:

1. Check national, state, and local laws before using your LED.
2. Avoid looking directly into the beam as it can cause a headache.
3. Make direct contact with the skin at all times or be as close as possible.

Contraindications of Light Therapy

Outside of the minor precautions regarding eye safety, there are a number of other precautions or contraindications. In spite of the fact that we have no documented evidence that the following problems will occur, it is better to be safe than sorry.

1. Do not treat over a known or suspected tumor or skin cancer. Although there has been no proof that this is dangerous, we do know that light therapy can stimulate the growth of many types of cells. However, in the field of oncology, light therapy is being used with many types of cancer patients to help manage pain and oral mucositis. If you are not sure if laser is appropriate, ask the patient's oncologist or physician.
2. Be cautious or avoid treatment during pregnancy. There has been no proof that light poses danger to pregnancy or pregnant women. Yet, due to the delicate nature of pregnancy and the natural possibilities for spontaneous abortion, a practitioner would be wise to avoid the use of light during pregnancy.

3. Photosensitivity reactions can occur because of many drugs, including antibiotics such as tetracycline, Retin-A, St. John's Wort, some thyroid medications, and possibly any medication with a warning to avoid bright sunlight.
4. Some practitioners believe that light should not be applied over the thyroid gland because iodine in the thyroid is a strong photo-absorber and could be stimulated by the laser. However, research indicates that low doses are quite safe.
5. Be cautious when treating over tattoos because dark-colored tattoos will absorb light and could become hot and painful.
6. Never treat directly over a bacterial infection. If you are treating an infected wound make sure the patient is on antibiotics and being monitored by a physician.
7. Do not treat patients on immune suppressant drugs since light therapy can stimulate the immune system and possibly interfere with the medical treatment.
8. Be careful treating children or sensitive adults. Always start with a very small total dose such as 25–50 joules for the first treatment.
9. Suspend therapy if the patient feels pain, weakness, or presents any other unusual reaction.

General Treatment Parameters

The treatment frequency or dose of treatment for Neuromusculoskeletal (NMS) syndromes and wounds depends on the severity of the syndrome. More acute problems require more frequent treatments. With chronic problems, the initial treatment needs a slightly lower dose than for acute injuries, and then also requires less frequent therapy:

Acute Syndromes: Treat 2 to 3 times per week until symptoms subside.

Subacute or Chronic Syndromes: Start with 2 times per week, followed by 1 to 2 times per week until symptoms have resolved.

Minimizing Adverse Side Effects: The 100 Joule Rule

Excessive light dosage can occasionally cause an adverse response.

1. If you are treating a very healthy, adult patient, the total treatment dose for the first session should not exceed 100 joules. With a very high powered LED, this may increase to 200 joules.
2. If the patient is suffering from any type of serious disorder, such as a non-healing wound or chronic pain, it is recommended that the first session utilize no more than 50 joules.

Treating Children: 50 Joule Rule

Use lower power and smaller doses when treating children. It is recommended that when treating children below the age of 12 years, to use an output of 50 joules or less during the first treatment, with a maximum of one-third to one-half the adult dosage, based on body weight.

Maximum Dose Depends on Power

1. Lower power LEDs (5 to 100 mW) require less total joules per treatment because they are more efficient and a higher percentage of the photons are absorbed by the tissues.
2. Higher power LEDs (1,000–10,000 mW) require more total joules because the large number of photons can produce heat and many of the photons are not utilized therapeutically.

Symptoms of Excessive Treatment

If the dose is too high, the patient may exhibit any of the following symptoms:

1. Muscular tightness
2. Mild fatigue or nausea
3. Pain or heat at the treatment site
4. Headache
5. An increase in symptom severity

These symptoms can occur during or after treatment and typically last from 1 to 48 hours.

Initial Treatment: 50% Rule

Assuming you are using a 1,000 mW device, it is safest to start an adult with no more than 100 joules on the first session and for a child, 50 joules. This dose can be increased as long as each successive dose is increased by no more than 50% each treatment. Thus, for adults, the first session would be 100 joules, the next session 150, etc. Obviously, this can be modified depending on the type of patient and/or condition.

See the section on page 22, Dark and Light Skin, for more information on how different variables can affect the first and subsequent doses. It is best to warn the patient of the possibility of some increase in discomfort, even though that is rare.

Optimal Dose for Each Patient

The optimal dose for each patient can vary. This can be judged in the following way:

1. Ask the patient to report any sensation during treatment.
2. A warming or tingling sensation or a lessening of the symptoms can be good signs.
3. An immediate increase in pain is a bad sign. Stop treatment immediately. Next time, lower the dose.
4. Look for an observable reduction in any swelling or inflammation.
5. Test the patient for improvement in functional capacity. Ask the patient to perform a movement that triggered pain before the treatment.
6. Palpate the treated area for reduced tenderness and increased tone.

Ask the patient to note any negative reactions or improvements in the 24-hour period following treatment.

Where to Start

Treat from the center of the body toward the periphery.

Stimulating the body's central processes will aid treatments to peripheral areas. For example, with lymphedema, stimulating the proximal regions of the leg will increase its physiological activity and prepare it for the increased fluids which will flow up the leg from the foot or foreleg. The same is true with manual lymph drainage, it is important to stimulate the proximal leg veins before sending more lymph into them from the foot and ankle.

Calculating the Output of Your LED in Joules

The following is the approximate delivered dose in joules per minute, based on the output power of the LED.

10,000 mW	=	600 joules / minute
5000 mW	=	300 joules / minute
3000 mW	=	180 joules / minute
2000 mW	=	120 joules / minute
1000 mW	=	60 joules / minute
500 mW	=	30 joules / minute
100 mW	=	6 joules / minute
10 mW	=	.6 joules / minute

Maximum Treatment Time

Your total treatment time will be dependent on the strength of your LED because treatment time is inversely proportional to the LED's total output power. The maximum recommended dose for the average patient is 100 to 600 joules; with an LED that is 1,000 to 10,000 mW. Although there are exceptions, mentioned in the clinical part of this manual, we will use that maximum dose for the calculations below:

A 10,000 mW LED will produce 600 joules per minute.

> 10 watts × 60 seconds = 600 joules per minute
>
> Maximum treatment time: .5–2 minutes depending on the condition

A 5000 mW LED would produce 300 joules per minute.

> 5 watts × 60 seconds = 300 joules per minute
>
> Maximum treatment time: 1–3 minutes depending on the condition

A 1000 mW LED would produce approximately 60 joules per minute.

> 1 × 60 seconds = 60 joules per minute
>
> Maximum treatment time: 2–10 minutes depending on the condition

Light Before Heat and After Ice

Because photons are absorbed by blood and water, diminishing their depth of penetration, it is recommended that you use light therapy before any heat and after ice. Because diathermy, ultrasound, and hot packs increase local blood flow, they would also increase local hemoglobin concentration, thus robbing the deeper structures of some photons.

Dark and Light Skin: The 25% Rule

Dark-skinned individuals have more melanin, the brown pigment that blocks out the sun. People from areas farther from the equator have lighter skin and those from the tropics have darker skin. It has been hypothesized that people who live in dark climates might have developed lighter-colored, more translucent skin, in order to help them absorb more of the sun's rays and therefore produce adequate amounts of vitamin D. It has been established that darker-skinned people are blessed with greater natural protection from the harmful sun rays and have a lower risk of skin cancer.

If you are striving for deep light penetration, it is important to increase the laser dose for a dark-skinned individual and decrease the dose by the same amount when treating a light-skinned individual. The more extreme the skin color, the more you will need to modify your dose.

Painting Technique

This technique involves moving a cluster of LEDs over the selected area of treatment about half the speed of ultra-sound, or about one inch (2.5 centimeters) every 2 seconds. The movement should be steady, to allow for well-distributed photoabsorption.

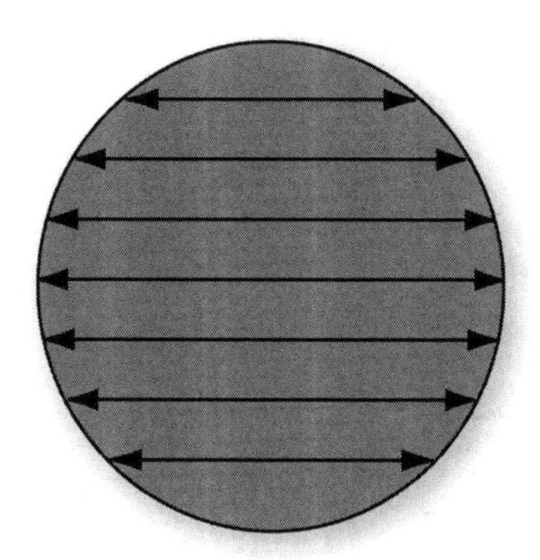

Nerve Tracing

Nerve tracing is used in cases with neuritis, sciatica, and radicu-lopathy. It involves palpation along the skin overlaying the tract of a peripheral nerve, looking for sore, tender points. Often the ten-der point is slightly raised, possibly indicating increased muscle tonus. The protocol would be:

1. Trace the nerve from proximal to distal.
2. Palpate the skin over a nerve looking for tender or swollen points.
3. Treat the most important tender points.

Hot and Cold Imbalance

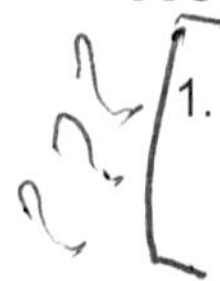

1. Stimulation of a cooler region with light can create increased warmth; stimulating a warmer region can create increased coolness.
2. This occurs because light has the ability to both stimulate and alter the autonomic nervous system, therefore stimulating natural homeostasis.

Relaxation Technique

1. When the probe is placed against the skin you will feel a certain amount of tissue resistance.
2. As you provide light stimulation you will, at some point, feel the device gently sink into the tissue.
3. This may reflect a relaxation response by the connective tissue.
4. This often means that the patient has received sufficient stimulation to relax tissues and is a sign to stop treatment on that particular point or region.

Treatment and Dosage Guidelines

1. For any one anatomical area, the lower dosages are better for stimulating healing and higher dosages will provide more pain relief.
2. For deeper areas, use the longer treatment time in the range but keep the device moving to avoid overheating and flaring the area.
3. If you want to treat 3 areas, use the lower part of the range for each area, but be careful not to over-treat.

4. With higher power LEDs in the range of 5,000–10,000 mW, extra caution needs to be exercised when treating multiple areas to avoid flaring up the patient.

You will find these charts at the beginning of each chapter of diagrams on pages 34, 52, 66, 82, and 102.

Head & Face Treatments

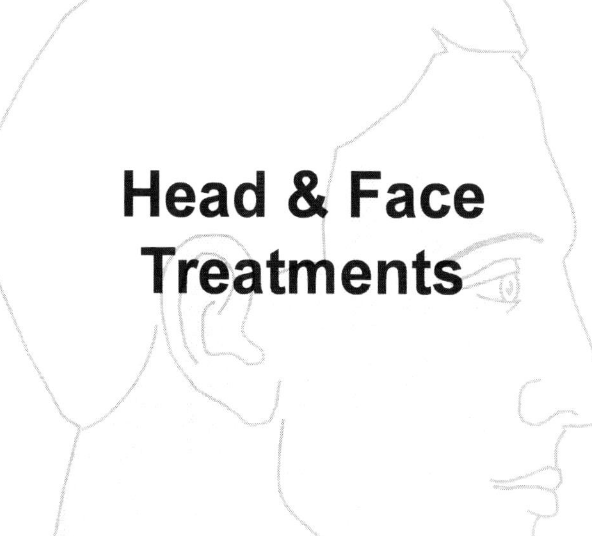

Bell's Palsy (diagram page 35, dose page 34)

Subjective: The patient will usually complain of an acute onset of unilateral upper and lower facial paralysis. This may be accompanied by ear pain, decreased hearing, occasionally hyperacusis and taste abnormalities. Onset may be insidious or after infection, trauma, or toxic exposure.

Assessment: The patient will often notice a decrease in discomfort, especially at night, after the first treatment.

Light Treatment Plan: Treatment can begin two to three times per week as long as symptoms are stable or improving. Begin by painting over the area of palsy as well as the course of the facial nerve with no more than 25 joules. Slowly increase dosage over the course of therapy with a maximum dose of 50 to 600 joules per treatment.

Adjunctive Treatment Plan: The patient should be educated about proper eye care and in facial exercise techniques. Taping the eye shut at night can make sleeping easier and protect the eye from injury.

Sinusitis (diagram page 38, dose page 34)

Subjective: Patients usually complain of chronic pain in and around one or more of the four sinuses in the frontal and maxillary bones. There may also be nasal stuffiness, the feeling of facial fullness, dental pain, fever, and ear pain.

Assessment: There will be a decrease in subjective complaints if inflammation and infection are alleviated.

Light Treatment Plan: Be certain that there is no infection prior to treating with laser therapy. If there is a significant amount of mucous, ask the patient to consult their doctor or start a saline flush before starting laser therapy. The mucous must be loose and draining before using a laser on the sinuses. Once the sinuses have started to drain, paint over the sinuses, starting with a total of 25–100 joules spread over the problematic sinuses, approximately 2 to 3 times per week. Intraoral irradiation into the maxillary sinus, radiation into the nostrils and treatment between the eyebrows can be of benefit. Only increase the dose if the patient is reporting an improvement in symptoms, and as long as the patient is using a saline wash.

Adjunctive Treatment Plan: Washing the sinuses with saline on a regular basis can be very helpful. Check environmental sensitivities or allergic factors as they may predispose some individuals to this condition. Ask the patient to reduce exposure to dust, molds, cigarette smoke, and irritants. In some cases, adding a mild herbal disinfectant to the saline flush or having a physician prescribe a liquid antibiotic from a compounding pharmacy can produce faster, more effective results.

Temporomandibular Joint (TMJ) Syndrome

(diagram page 39, dose page 34)

Subjective: Patients typically complain of pain in and around the TMJ. There is often increased pain with chewing, occasional popping and clicking. Many patients also complain of earache, headache, and limitation of jaw movement.

Assessment: Improvement is observed as decreased subjective complaints, less muscle spasm, with improving range of jaw motion.

Light Treatment Plan: Treat the masseter, pterygoids, and temporalis muscles. Rarely does the joint need more than 10 to 100 joules, but the muscles do require a stronger dose. Begin with 25 joules on the first treatment and, with a higher power LED, titrate up to a maximum of 600 joules if condition shows improvement with each increase.

Adjunctive Treatment Plan: The use of ice and heat is recommended to control inflammation and pain. Educate the patient about bruxism, tongue and jaw position, and the need to avoid clenching. Stress can play a major role in the disturbance of jaw posture and thus stress reduction strategies and behavior modification can be of benefit. Good posture, soft food, and smaller bites can make eating easier. If treatment is ineffective a splint to stabilize the TMJ is another option.

Tension and Migraine Headaches

(diagrams pages 36–37, dose page 34)

Subjective: Tension headaches are characterized by a generalized aching that tends to be experienced as a constant pressure in the frontal, temporal, and occipital regions. Migraines often have a prodrome and are very severe compared to tension headaches. Many patients state that stress, eyestrain, bad posture, and hunger can aggravate their condition.

Assessment: Since lab and imaging studies only rule out pathology and are not diagnostic, patient history and pain level are utilized to asses improvement after treatment. Tight muscles in neck and face should decrease.

Light Treatment Plan: Deliver 100–200 joules to the area of discomfort, primarily the suboccipital and upper cervical regions. Follow this with painting of the frontal or temporalis muscles if pain is also present in those regions.

Adjunctive Treatment Plan: The use of ice and heat is recommended to control inflammation and pain. Additional techniques include cervical stretching exercises, massage, ultrasound therapy, and cranial and cervical spine mobilization. Some patients find benefit from meditation, stress management, and biofeedback techniques. For migraines, medication is often necessary.

Weight Loss and Body Contouring

(dose page 34)

Subjective: The patient complains of difficulty losing weight.

Assessment: Girth and weight should show a slow reduction with time.

Light Treatment Plan: If you have a powerful LED, like 5,000 – 10,000 milliwatts, you will treat the area for about 2 minutes.

Adjunctive Treatment Plan: There is a significant amount of research that substantiates using light therapy as an adjunct to other weight loss measures like proper diet, portion control, and exercise. Studies show that adding light therapy to areas of heavy fat deposition may make dieting and exercise more successful. It is thought that light therapy may improve the body's ability to rid itself of fat in adipose cells.

Wrinkles (dose page 34)

Subjective: Patient presents with a desire for a smoother facial complexion.

Objective: The size and depth of lines can be measured, although typically patients are very aware of their facial contours and can report quite accurately if treatment is making a difference.

Assessment: Patient and therapist can observe a lessened number of the shallower wrinkles.

Light Treatment Plan: Start treating with 50 to 100 joules the first visit and increase to 200–600 joules if there are no side effects and patient is happy with the results. It could take one to two months of treatment, 2 to 3 times per week, to produce a significant change.

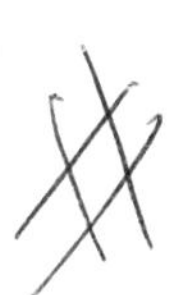

Adjunctive Treatment Plan: Make sure the patient is using a quality moisturizing cream after each treatment. Some therapists report that supplementing the treatment with oral hyaluronic acid and essential fatty acids can increase the speed and quality of improvement.

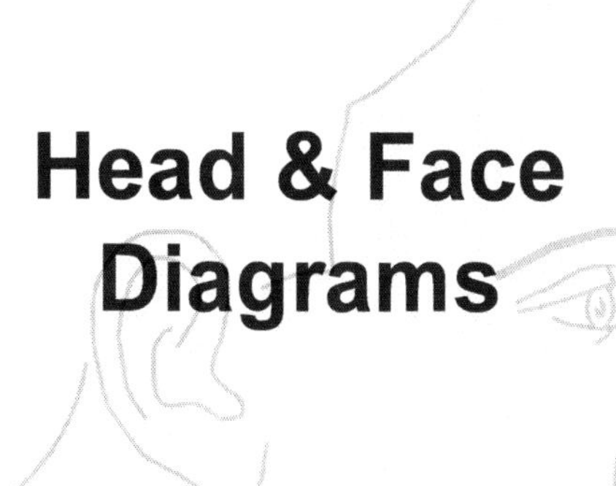

Head & Face Diagrams

Typical Treatment Time and Joules based on Power of Device

Probe Output (mW)	Joules	Treatment Time
10	6 - 12	10 - 20 mins
100	36 - 72	6 - 12 mins
500	60 - 180	2 - 6 mins
1,000	90 - 240	1.5 - 4 mins
2,000	120 - 360	1 - 3 mins
4,000	240 - 480	1 - 2 mins
6,000	270 - 540	.75 - 1.5 mins
8,000	240 - 600	.5 - 1.25 mins
10,000	150 - 600	.25 - 1 min

The above chart notes the approximate treatment times based on the power of the device being used. Since the suggested treatment doses in this book are for LEDs in the range of 10 to 10,000 mW, full body treatment times will be approximately 1–15 minutes and approximately 100 to 1200 joules. If you are using a lower power LED, you will need to use longer treatment times, and proportionally less joules.

Use this chart as a guide for an approximate treatment time and dosage based on your particular LED and the individual needs of the patient.

Bell's Palsy

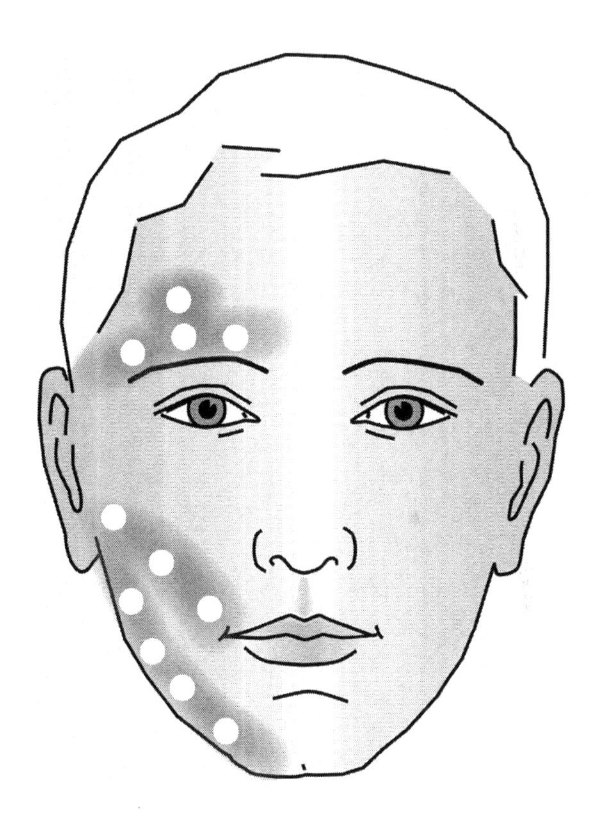

Headache

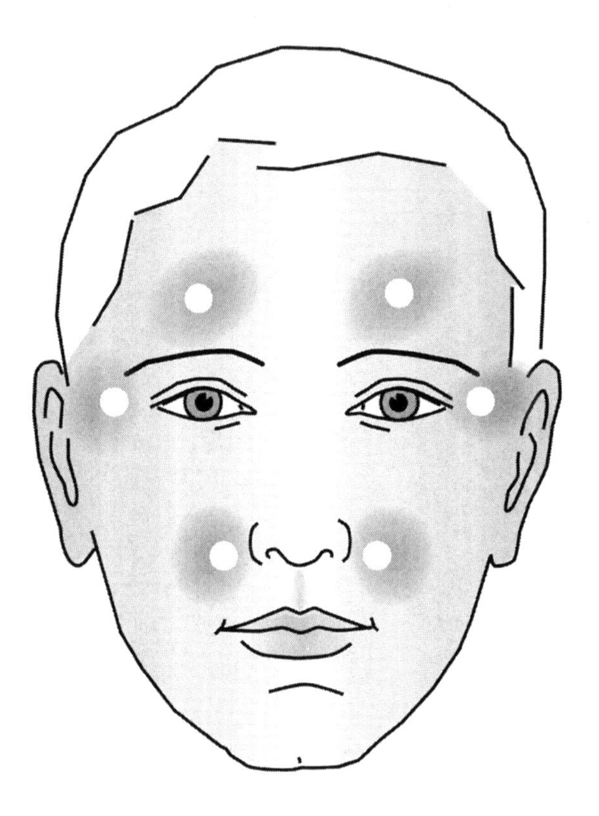

Headache

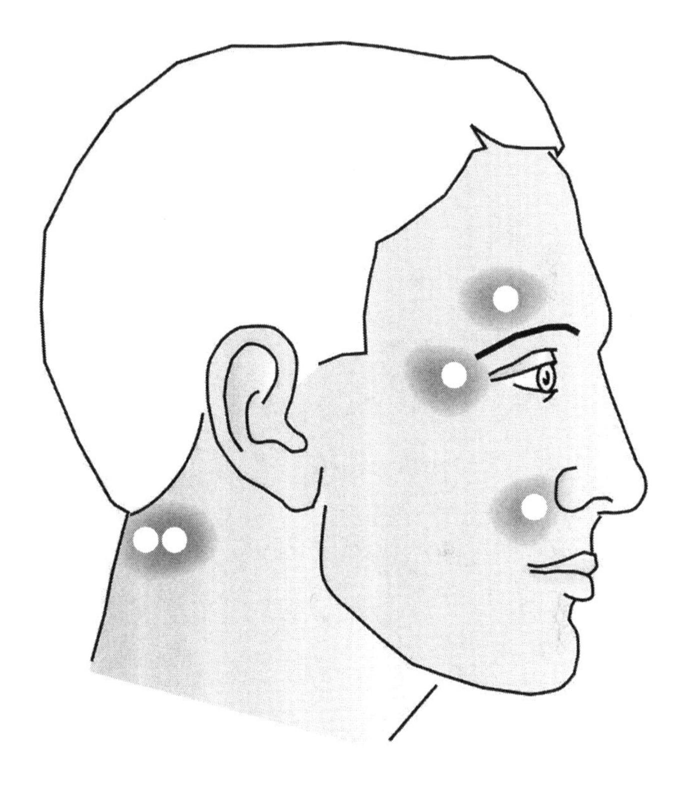

Sinusitis

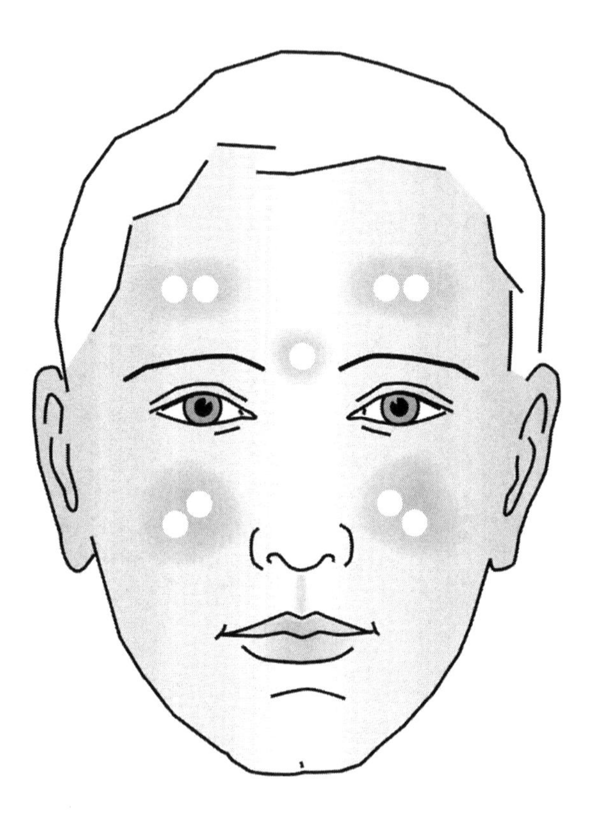

TMJ Syndrome

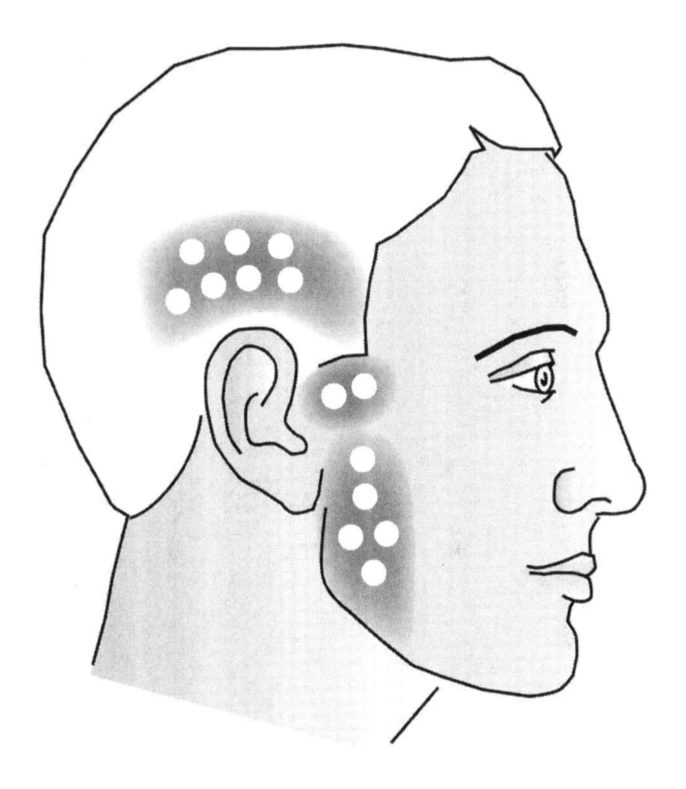

Trigeminal Neuralgia

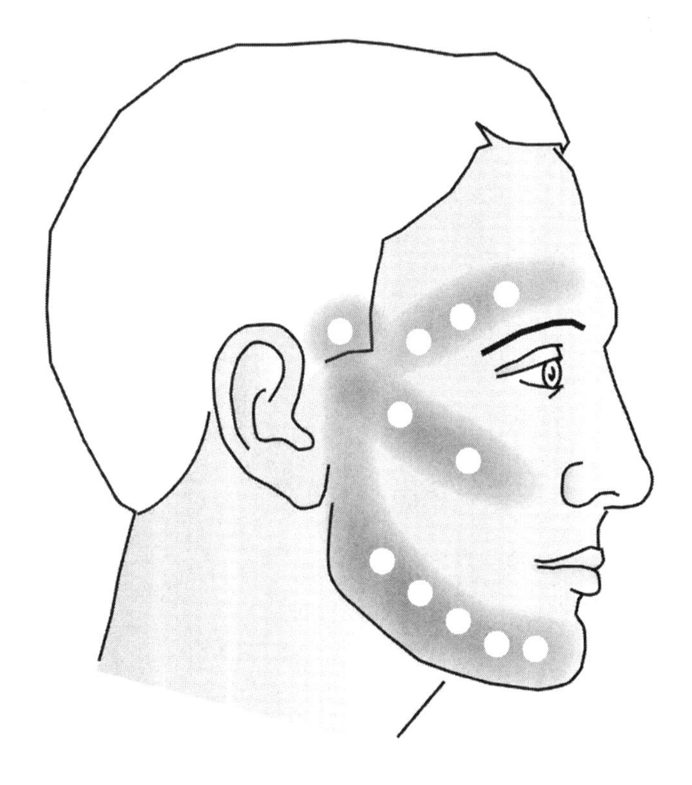

Spine & Pelvis Treatments

Cervical Disc Herniation and Stenosis

(diagram page 54, dose page 52)

Subjective: Herniated cervical discs create pain in the lateral neck and shoulder in mild cases. In moderate to serious cases, there can be severe pain that radiates into the ipsilateral middle back, arm and hand. The patient may present a history of trauma, but insidious onset is common.

Assessment: Improvement will result in centralization of pain followed by decreasing neck pain, increasing range of motion, and, when present, normalizing neurological signs.

Light Treatment Plan: Treat the site of herniation with 25–600 joules and then slowly paint over the nerve roots in the lateral neck with 10 to 100 joules. Finally, trace a few tender points in the arm with 5 to 25 joules per tender point. Treat two to three times per week for two to six weeks, decreasing frequency as symptoms improve.

Adjunctive Treatment Plan: Most patients find relief from avoiding cervical spine extension and ipsilateral side bending. Many patients report relief from gentle home traction and regular resting in the supine position, to minimize loading of the disc. Prescribe arm and chest stretches to relieve brachial tension, with an emphasis on middle back strengthening as symptoms abate. Initial use of ice and then later use of ice/heat on the cervical spine can be helpful to decrease inflammation and control symptoms. A home program that includes upper extremity stretching can be helpful. If symptoms are not improving after two to three weeks, or if there is increasing pain or motor weakness, consider a referral to an orthopedic specialist.

Cervical, Thoracic, Lumbar Sprain/Strain

(diagram page 53, dose page 52)

Subjective: Sprains and strains typically cause localized back or neck pain. In moderate cases, there will be muscle spasm and even radiating pain into an extremity or around the ribs and into the chest or abdomen, especially with moderate injuries to facets or ribs. The patient may feel relief with flexion or extension.

Assessment: With appropriate therapy, the patient will note improved joint play with decreasing spasm and pain within the first few treatments.

Light Treatment Plan: Treat two to three times the first week, decreasing frequency as symptoms subside. Treat with 10 to 100 joules directly over the problem facet. Treat with 5 to 25 joules per tender point if there is radiating pain down the arm, leg, or along intercostal nerves if there is a radiating neuritis. Maximum initial dose should not exceed 100 to 150 joules, increasing to a maximum of 600 joules per session.

Adjunctive Treatment Plan: In the acute stage, the patient should avoid any position or movement that increases pain. Initially using ice for 2 to 3 days and then ice/heat can assist in symptom control. Mobilization often provides dramatic relief of symptoms. Patient should only perform exercises that provide relief from pain in early stages and progress to gentle stretching and strengthening as symptoms decrease. With rib sprains, no flexion or side-bending stretching should be performed for one to two days after joint mobilization. If one week of treatment has not produced significant improvement, consider referral to an orthopedic specialist for more potent anti-inflammatories and an additional diagnostic workup.

Coccydynia (diagram page 54, dose page 52)

Subjective: Patients usually complain of lower coccyx pain that is aggravated by sitting. Although onset can be insidious, the most common cause is direct trauma or repeated strain caused by activities such as cycling or rowing. Childbirth, due to the increased flexibility of the joint and the resulting strain and pressure, can also cause this syndrome. The result is an injury of the sacrococcygeal junction.

Assessment: Improvement will be noted after 1–2 weeks as a decrease in localized, sacrococcygeal complaints. If improvement is interrupted by a flare-up, make certain that the patient uses upright and slightly forward leaning posture when sitting.

Light Treatment Plan: Begin treatment with 25 to 100 joules with half of the treatment painting directly over the sacrococcygeal junction and the other half slowly painting the adjacent areas of the sacrum and gluteal muscles.

Adjunctive Treatment Plan: To reduce direct strain on the coccyx, patients need to be encouraged to avoid sitting down for long periods of time. Sitting on the edge of the chair, with the weight on the ischial tuberosities, can often reduce pain over time. Some practitioners believe that intra-anal mobilization techniques may be of benefit. Anti-inflammatories, ice, and sitting on a "doughnut" cushion or pillow can help control symptoms. In acute cases a stool softener can reduce discomfort during defecation.

Costochondritis or Chest Pain

(diagram page 53, dose page 52)

Subjective: This condition often presents with sternal or rib pain localized to the costal cartilage. This syndrome is common after motor vehicle accidents and sports injuries, but can be of insidious onset.

Assessment: Treatment usually results in rapid resolution of the majority of symptoms.

Light Treatment Plan: Treat each tender sternocostal joint with 10 to 50 joules and then paint over the wider symptomatic area with 25 to 100 joules. Treatment in the acute stage often requires no more than two to five treatments, each with a maximum of 50 to 600 joules.

Adjunctive Treatment Plan: Ice/heat at home can help reduce inflammation. Stretching should be avoided for one to two days after treatment. Gentle mobilization of the sternocostal and costovertebral joints can help alleviate dysfunction, when present.

Herniated Lumbar Disc

(diagram page 54, dose page 52)

Subjective: A herniated lumbar disc will create low back and/or leg pain that is increased with at least one or two of the following activities: coughing, sneezing, sitting, long term standing, rolling over in bed, moving from lying or sitting to standing, and repeated bending, twisting, and lifting.

Assessment: Proper therapy usually results in improving range of motion, decreased pain, and less positive orthopedic tests.

Light Treatment Plan: On the first treatment, start with 25–600 joules depending upon the severity of the injury. Always start with a lower dose and titrate upward slowly. Treat two to three times the first week, decreasing frequency as symptoms improve. Use lower doses if patient has severe pain, to reduce the likelihood of a flare-up. Spend one-third of the treatment time directly over the injured disc, one-third painting the lumbar nerve roots above and across the crest of the ilium, and one-third of the dose treating points in the buttocks and leg. Treatment may be required over the lumbar or leg muscles if there is spasm, including hamstrings, quadratus lumborum, gluteus medius, and tensor fascia lata.

Adjunctive Treatment Plan: In the acute stage, the patient should decrease sitting, bending, twisting, and lifting. Initially using ice and then ice/heat can assist in symptom control. A back brace often provides an increased sense of stability during the most acute stage. The patient should only perform exercises that provide relief from pain in early stages and progress to stabilization exercises and leg stretching as symptoms decrease. Later, progression to stabilization and strengthening of core muscles is recommended. Traction can be provided when appropriate, and education about posture and body mechanics is vital.

If there is no improvement after one to two weeks or symptoms worsen, a referral to an orthopedic specialist may be indicated for an MRI or other types of intervention. If there is bladder or bowel disruption or a noticeable increase in neurological symptoms, especially motor weakness, refer the patient to a physician immediately.

Lumbar Stenosis (diagram page 54, dose page 52)

Subjective: Lumbar stenosis commonly presents with low back pain that radiates into the hip and lower extremity, aggravated by lumbar spine extension. Often lying prone aggravates the pain, while slumped sitting and pelvic tilt positions can give some relief.

Assessment: If treatment is successful, the patient will experience less radiating pain and improved functional activities.

Light Treatment Plan: Treat the site of stenosis with 25 to 200 joules and then paint over the nerve roots with 10 to 100 joules above the crest of the ilium. Finally, trace the radiating pain down the sciatic nerve with 5 to 25 joules per tender point with treatment of the foot and toenails in severe cases, for a maximum of 50 to 600 joules per session.

Adjunctive Treatment Plan: Initial use of ice and then later use of ice/heat on the lumbar spine can be helpful to decrease inflammation and control symptoms. A home program that includes application of heat to the leg muscles and lower extremity stretching can also be helpful. Most patients find relief from gentle flexion exercises, leg stretches, with an emphasis on abdominal and core strengthening. If symptoms are not improving after two to three weeks, or if there is increasing pain or motor weakness, consider an immediate referral to an orthopedic specialist.

Pubic Symphysis Sprain

(diagram page 54, dose page 52)

Subjective: This syndrome will create pain at the pubic symphysis, aggravated by activity, even walking. In more severe cases, patients can hear a "clicking" emanating from the joint with vigorous physical activity, trauma, pregnancy, or obesity.

Assessment: With improvement, there is a rapid decrease in subjective complaints.

Light Treatment Plan: Place the probe directly over the most painful part of the pubic bones for 10 to 100 joules. Then paint over the area with 25 to 50 joules. Treatment can be provided two to three times per week for one to three weeks, decreasing frequency of treatment as symptoms abate. Because the symphysis is close to the genitals, consider having the patient hold the probe over the pubis.

Adjunctive Treatment Plan: Initial use of ice and then later use of ice/heat can be helpful to decrease inflammation and control symptoms. Patients should avoid any extreme range of motion of the lower extremities. Isometric thigh adduction and abduction can strengthen and stabilize the region once the acute symptoms have been relieved. In some cases, mobilization or stabilization of the sacroiliac joint can help alleviate pubic symptoms.

Sacroiliac Sprain (diagram page 53, dose page 52)

Subjective: A sacroiliac sprain or strain will create low back pain that centers primarily over the PSIS (posterior superior iliac spine) with, in more serious cases, pain radiation down the lateral thigh, but above the knee. Pain can sometimes be relieved by sitting and aggravated by walking or repeated bending and twisting.

Assessment: Decreased localized pain with increased range of motion.

Light Treatment Plan: Place the probe over the superior and the inferior part of the joint to deliver 25 to 100 joules per region. Painting over the joint and treatment of tender points in the gluteal region and the lateral thigh may help reduce symptoms. Treat two to three times, over a period of one to two weeks, or until symptoms have significantly decreased. Utilize a maximum of 50–600 joules per session.

Adjunctive Treatment Plan: Mobilization can often provide rapid, short-term relief. Initial use of ice and then later use of ice/heat can be helpful to decrease inflammation and control symptoms. Patient should only perform gentle exercises that provide relief from pain in early stages. Often, active and passive hip flexion and extension exercises can "self-mobilize" the joint and provide relief. In the subacute stage, progress to stabilization exercises and strengthening of core muscles. If one week of treatment has not produced significant improvement, consider referral to an orthopedic specialist.

Spine & Pelvis Diagrams

Typical Treatment Time and Joules based on Power of Device

Probe Output (mW)	Joules	Treatment Time
10	6 - 12	10 - 20 mins
100	36 - 72	6 - 12 mins
500	60 - 180	2 - 6 mins
1,000	90 - 240	1.5 - 4 mins
2,000	120 - 360	1 - 3 mins
4,000	240 - 480	1 - 2 mins
6,000	270 - 540	.75 - 1.5 mins
8,000	240 - 600	.5 - 1.25 mins
10,000	150 - 600	.25 - 1 min

The above chart notes the approximate treatment times based on the power of the device being used. Since the suggested treatment doses in this book are for LEDs in the range of 10 to 10,000 mW, full body treatment times will be approximately 1–15 minutes and approximately 100 to 1200 joules. If you are using a lower power LED, you will need to use longer treatment times, and proportionally less joules.

Use this chart as a guide for an approximate treatment time and dosage based on your particular LED and the individual needs of the patient.

Spine & Pelvis

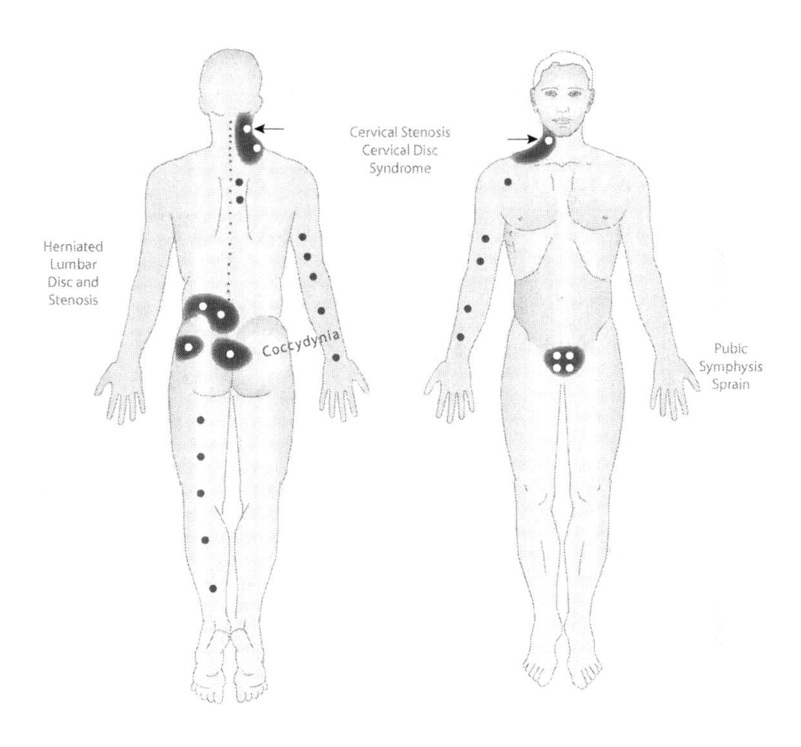

Spine & Pelvis

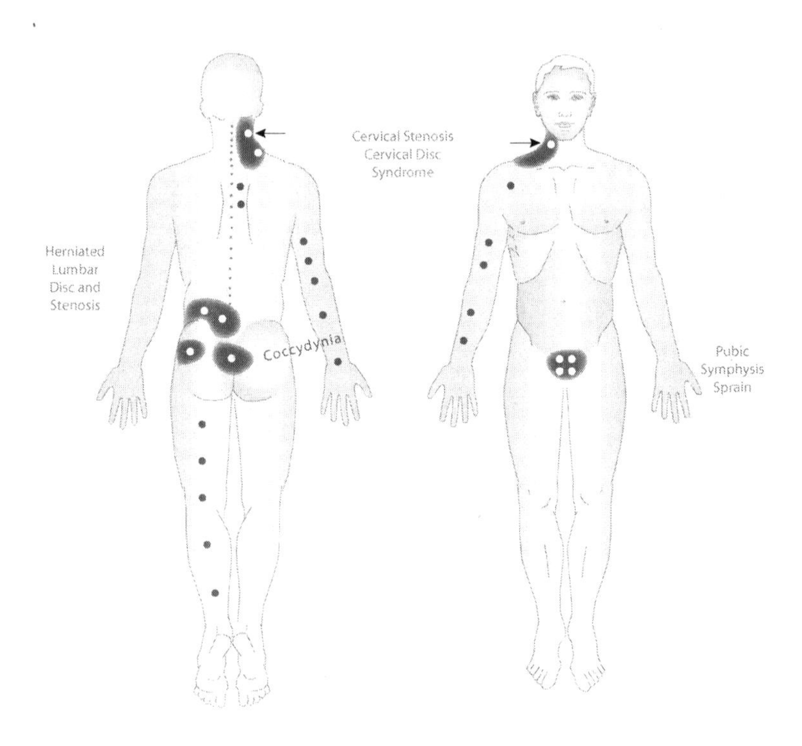

Systemic Treatments

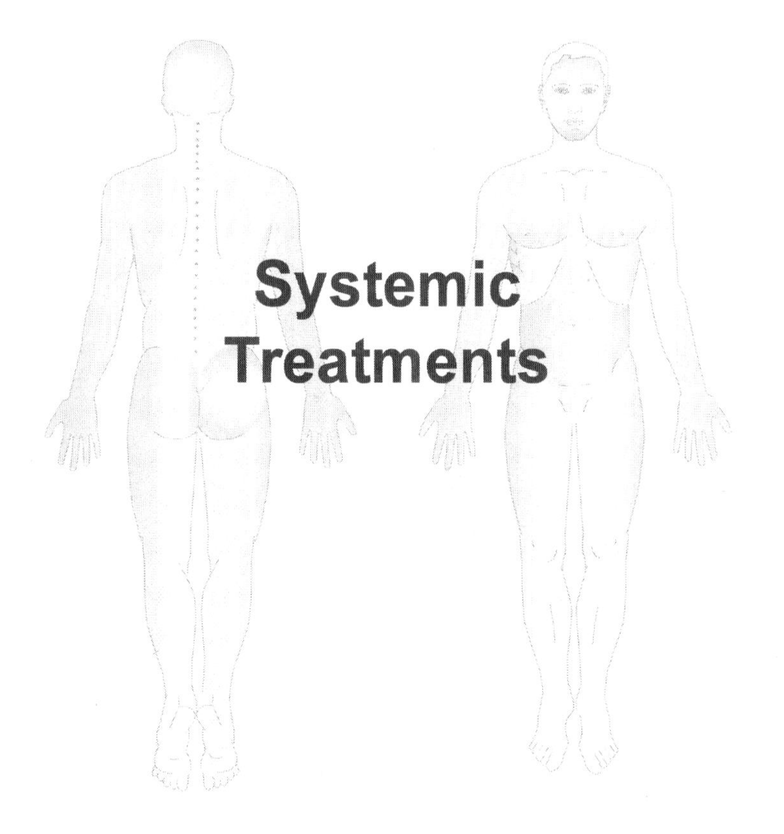

Arthritis (diagram page 68, dose page 78)

See individual syndromes for more specific treatments of different types of arthritis.

Subjective: There will be swelling, stiffness, and pain. Symptoms may be worse in the morning.

Assessment: There will be a decrease in swelling and pain. However, with more severe rheumatoid arthritis, light will manage symptoms but will not provide a lasting cure.

Light Treatment Plan: Treat most areas with 5 to 25 joules points per point, with smaller joints receiving a total of 25 to 50 joules and larger joints 50 to 600 joules. Remember to treat all four sides of the joint. To improve depth of penetration, place the device on one spot without moving it. Osteoarthritis seems to respond better than rheumatoid arthritis.

Hands/Fingers: Treat smaller joints like fingers and toes with less joules than larger joints such as the knee and hip. Measure improvement by decrease in stiffness and swelling, pain-free motion, and measuring grip strength with a pinch gauge or dynamometer.

Wrist: Treat around the circumference of the joint with special attention to the primary area of pain.

Elbow: Identify areas of tenderness, and treat over the lateral and medial epicondyles as well as the adjacent soft tissue.

Shoulder: Causes may be multifactorial, involving the shoulder, acromioclavicular and sternoclavicular joints, muscles, tendons, ligaments, and bursae.

TMJ: Make certain that you treat the TMJ and the adjacent muscles.

Hip: The most efficient access to the acetabulum is best accomplished from the groin (anterior acetabulum) and sciatic notch.

Knee: Soft tissues around the knee, such as the subpatellar and suprapatellar tendon and ligaments, respond more quickly than problems deep within the joint.

Ankle: It is important to treat the area where the problem resides, such as the subtalar or talocrural joint.

Foot/Toes: Smaller joints such as the fingers and toes usually require no more than 25 to 50 joules per joint. With smaller joints and a larger cluster device, many of the photons are lost because of the poor alignment between the device and the rounded joint structure.

Adjunctive Treatment Plan: Gentle stretching and range of motion activities are beneficial. Some patients find improvement in symptoms with a combination of oral glucosamine sulfate and MSM (methylsulfonylmethane).

Bursitis (dose page 66)

Subjective: The patient complains of pain and decreased range of motion due to a swollen bursa. A bursa is the small, fluid-filled sac that can cushion the tendons and muscles near your joints. The most common areas for bursitis are the shoulder, elbow, and hip. But they can also occur in the knee, heel, and the base of the big toe.

Assessment: With treatment, the area of pain will decrease and pain-free range of motion will increase.

Shoulder: The most common bursitis is the subacromial bursa. It is just beneath the acromion process of the clavicle and the rotator cuff muscles and tendons. Treat with friction massage, stretching, ice and 1–2 minutes of light therapy.

Hip: The greater trochanteric bursa is the most common site of hip bursitis. It covers the greater trochanter can create pain with walking. Treat with gentle massage, stretching, ice, and 1–2 minutes of light therapy.

Elbow: The posterior tip of the elbow is the site of olecranon bursitis. It can swell to resemble part of a golf ball and can require medical care if it becomes infected. Treat with ice and 1–2 minutes of light therapy.

Knee: The most common sites are: 1. Prepatellar bursitis, just below the kneecap (Housemaid's Knee), 2. Semimembranosis bursitis which is in the back of the knee (Baker's Cyst), and 3. Infrapatellar bursitis, which is just below the kneecap.

Light Treatment Plan: Use 1–2 minutes of light therapy if you have a powerful LED. If you have a low power LED, it could take 15–20 minutes. Use mild pressure to get photons deep into the bursa.

Adjunctive Treatment Plan: Use 5 minutes of ice before light therapy for the first few days. Then add gentle massage. If the swelling worsens and turns red and inflamed, you may need a physician to rule out the need for antibiotics or draining the fluid with aspiration.

Complex Regional Pain Syndrome or Reflex Sympathetic Dystrophy

(diagram page 69, dose page 66)

Subjective: RSD or CRPS is a very painful syndrome that can cause swelling, redness, temperature changes, and moderate to severe pain. It usually occurs in the hands or feet, although it can occur almost anywhere in the body. The cause of the pain is often due to a minor trauma that surprisingly creates this serious pain condition.

Assessment: There will be a decrease in pain and an associated normalizing of temperature in the symptomatic limb.

Light Treatment Plan: Treatment can be given two to three times a week for up to three or four weeks to see if light therapy can be of benefit. It is important to start treatment with a very low dose and only increase the dose slowly and carefully, once positive results appear. Positive effects include a decrease in pain and temperature change of one or all of the limbs. Negative effects can be an increase in pain. The first treatment should be no more than 10 to 20 total joules, only increasing if there is no increase in pain.

Start by treating along the transverse processes of the thoracic spine (C7 to L2). This correlates with the sympathetic chain ganglia (SCG). If this does not produce any positive effects, try giving the next treatment to the stellate ganglia (SG), which is located on the anterior lateral transverse process of the seventh cervical vertebra. If symptoms are improved or there is no change, in the next session treat the SCG or the SG with a slightly higher dose, such as 20 to 100 joules. If symptoms are improved or there is no change, in the next session treat the SCG and the SG. If treating the SCG and the SG produces no side effects, try treating the opposite limb and assess if there is any improvement in symptoms. Only treat the symptomatic limb once treatment has been directed to the SCG, SG, and then opposite limb over a series of treatments with no negative side effects or some mild decrease in symptoms.

Adjunctive Treatment Plan: Medical management is imperative and light therapy must be performed with the approval or supervision of a physician. Range-of-motion stretching, medication, nutritional counseling, and gentle cardiovascular exercise are vital in maintaining the health of the injured limb.

Fibromyalgia Syndrome (diagram page 70, dose page 66)

Subjective: Most patients complain of morning stiffness and sleep problems. Many complain of feeling as if they have swollen extremities, with numbness and tingling. These symptoms generally are more common in the upper than in the lower extremities.

Assessment: Improvement is slow and steady.

Light Treatment Plan: Treat with no more than 25 joules the first treatment, composed of 5 to 10 joules per point. Later, with improving symptoms, dose can be increased to a total full body dose of 50 to 600 joules as long as it is titrated slowly.

Adjunctive Treatment Plan: A multidisciplinary treatment plan composed of exercise combined with education and cognitive behavioral therapy can be highly effective. In addition, gentle manipulation and massage can help decrease stiffness and pain. Daily aerobic and flexibility exercises should be performed at least three times weekly starting gently and slowly increasing in intensity. Warm water aquatic therapy is well tolerated and especially helpful for some patients.

Herpes, Shingles, and Postherpetic Neuralgia (diagram page 67, dose page 66)

Subjective: Patients complain initially of a small area of painful, red lesions. Over time the severity of pain usually increases and can become severe.

Assessment: Initially there will be a decrease in pain followed by the disappearance of the lesions.

Light Treatment Plan: Treatments twice weekly for three weeks are appropriate for acute cases, followed by once per week after there has been a significant decrease in pain. Utilize a maximum of 25 to 100 joules on the first visit.

Adjunctive Treatment Plan: A referral to a physician for antiviral medication or herbs, laboratory testing, or imaging studies may be necessary in more serious cases.

Postsurgical Pain

Subjective: Pain in the area of the surgery.

Assessment: Pain will be reduced within hours and should create less need for analgesics and anti-inflammatories.

Light Treatment Plan: First treatment is 25 to 50 joules over the average size wound surface. Raise the dose slowly if there is positive response.

Adjunctive Treatment Plan: Icing the area prior to treatment can assist in the reduction of inflammation.

Wounds (Slow or Non-Healing)

(diagram page 67, dose page 66)

Subjective: Patients report impaired healing of wounds. The problem is more common in diabetics and those with circulation difficulties. Make certain that the patient does not have the obvious signs of infection, including fever higher than 100°F, significant pain, increasing redness or faint red lines, heat, chills, lymph swelling or tenderness, pus, or swelling. If there is any suspicion that the wound is infected, refer the patient to a physician immediately.

Assessment: The initial goal is to decrease discomfort. The size of the wound will decrease with time as the perimeter begins to heal. Watch for possible signs of infection and refer the patient to a physician if this is suspected.

Light Treatment Plan: Treatment is ideal after the wound has been cleaned, as the presence of thick, poor-quality tissue will attenuate the absorption of the light beam.

The most common method is to treat the wound by "painting" back and forth over the wound with a cluster of LEDs. A wound that is 2.5 cm (1 inch) in diameter would need an initial dose of approximately 25 to 100 joules. Treatment can commence daily with decreasing frequency as the wound begins to close and heal. Spend two-thirds of the treatment time on the periphery where there is a higher concentration of actively dividing cells and one-third of the time on the center of the wound where more of the cells are less active. This is done to most effectively stimulate cell growth and improve healing.

If you are using a device designed to treat acupuncture and trigger points, it is more effective to treat a grid of points that covers the wound. However, it is still important to deliver more of the photons to the periphery than the center of the wound.

Patients may experience an immediate decrease or an increase in pain. Treating with a low dose on the first treatment and then titrating upward with each subsequent session can minimize this reaction.

It is most effective to treat the wound with laser when changing a bandage or dressing. However, it is not imperative to take the bandage off the wound before treating. Using a red or IR device, it is possible to treat in contact with the sterile dressing. However, you will need to double or triple the dosage because a typical gauze bandage significantly reduces the number of photons passing into the wound.

Wounds can be treated up to two to three times a week, decreasing frequency as the wound heals. It is common for more critical wounds to require 20 visits or more. Less serious wounds can respond after five to ten treatments. Occasional treatments may be necessary afterwards to continue promoting tissue regeneration and complete wound resolution.

Studies show that higher doses are more analgesic and lower doses stimulate healing more effectively. Thus, if healing plateaus before resolution, consider increasing or decreasing the dose to a maximum of 600 joules with a high power probe.

Adjunctive Treatment Plan: Be certain that the wound is not infected by making sure that the physician supervising the treatment is a specialist in wound care. Make sure that the patient has an excellent diet and the wound is cleaned frequently.

Systemic Diagrams

Typical Treatment Time and Joules based on Power of Device

Probe Output (mW)	Joules	Treatment Time
10	6 - 12	10 - 20 mins
100	36 - 72	6 - 12 mins
500	60 - 180	2 - 6 mins
1,000	90 - 240	1.5 - 4 mins
2,000	120 - 360	1 - 3 mins
4,000	240 - 480	1 - 2 mins
6,000	270 - 540	.75 - 1.5 mins
8,000	240 - 600	.5 - 1.25 mins
10,000	150 - 600	.25 - 1 min

The above chart notes the approximate treatment times based on the power of the device being used. Since the suggested treatment doses in this book are for LEDs in the range of 10 to 10,000 mW, full body treatment times will be approximately 1–15 minutes and approximately 100 to 1200 joules. If you are using a lower power LED, you will need to use longer treatment times, and proportionally less joules.

Use this chart as a guide for an approximate treatment time and dosage based on your particular LED and the individual needs of the patient.

Systemic

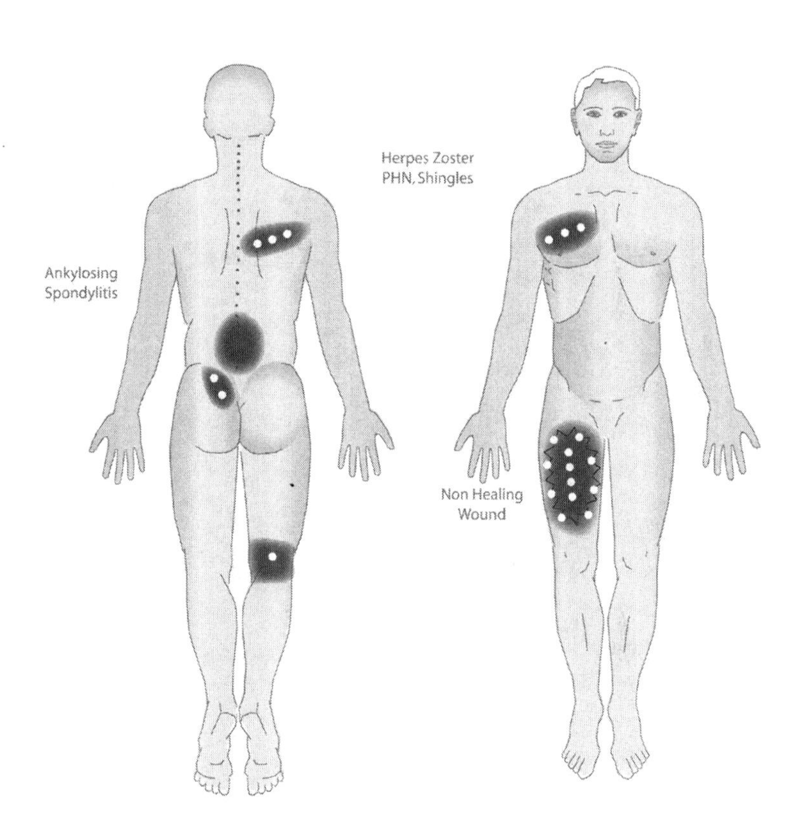

Herpes Zoster
PHN, Shingles
Ankylosing
Spondylitis
Non Healing
Wound

Arthritis

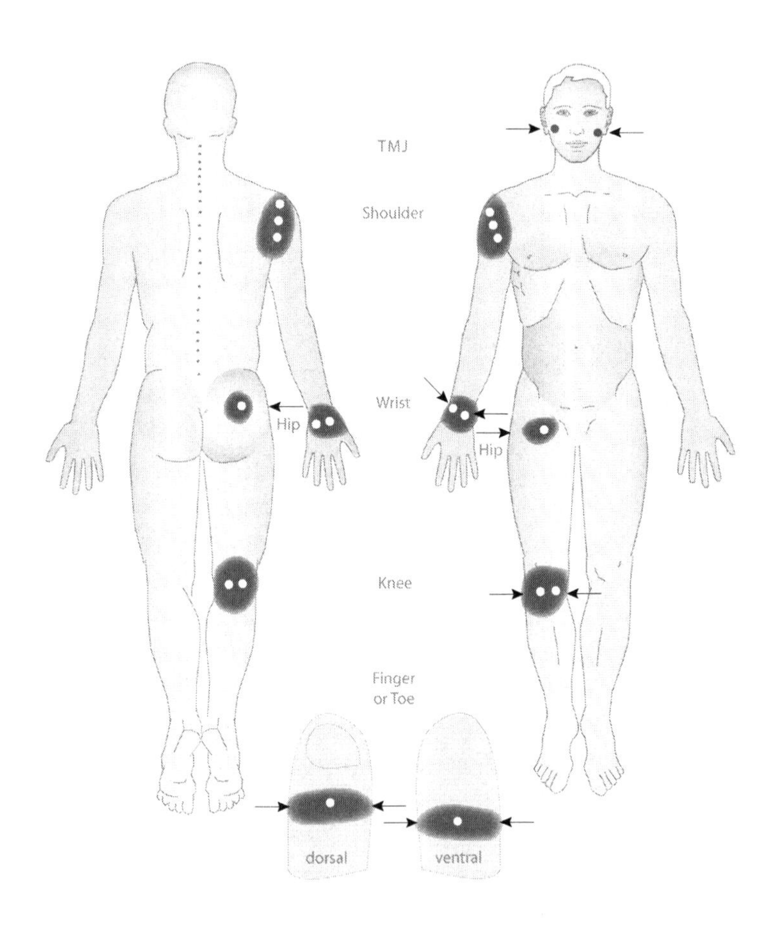
TMJ
Shoulder
Wrist
Hip
Hip
Knee
Finger
or Toe
dorsal
ventral

CRPS

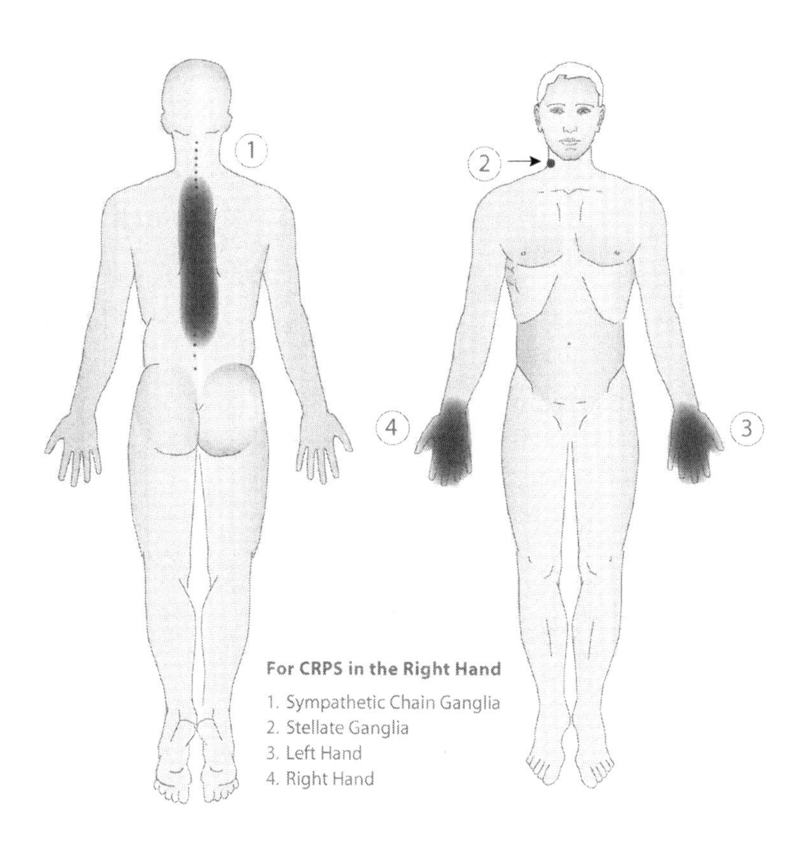
1
2
4
3
For CRPS in the Right Hand
1. Sympathetic Chain Ganglia
2. Stellate Ganglia
3. Left Hand
4. Right Hand

Fibromyalgia

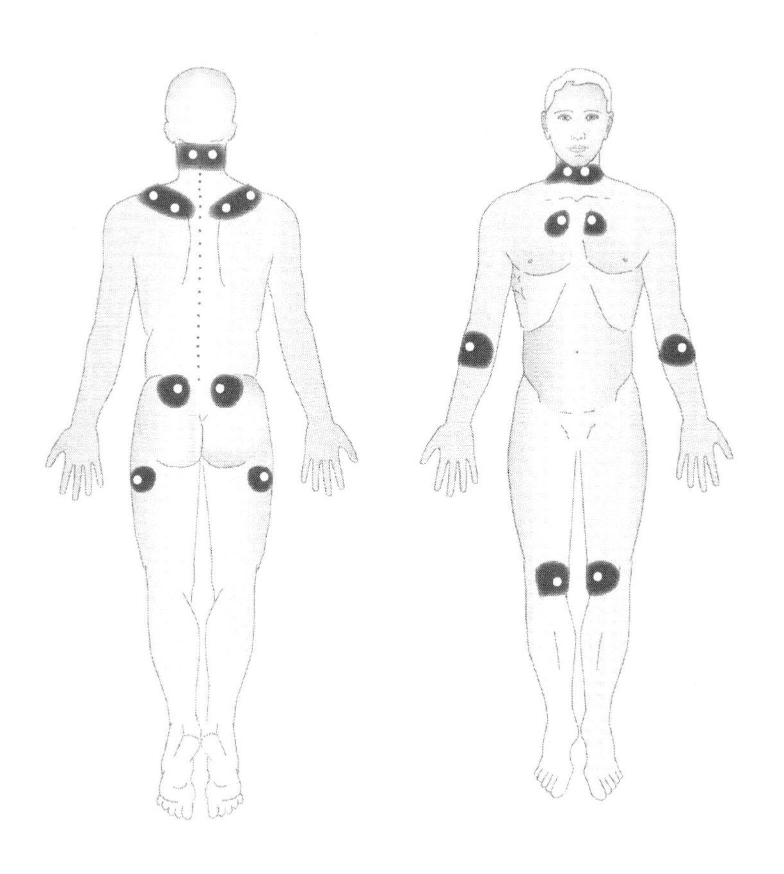

Upper Body Treatments

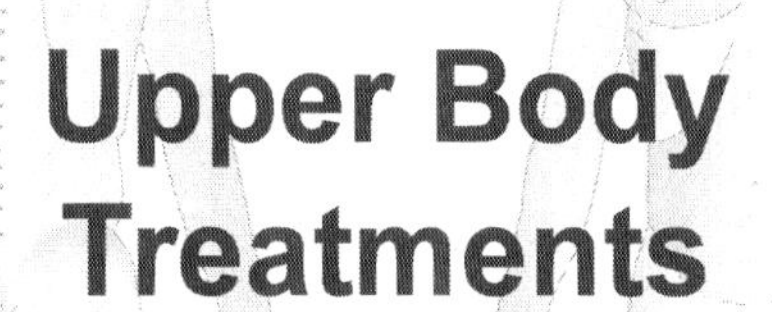

Biceps Tendinitis or Strain

(diagram page 83, dose page 82)

Subjective: Pain in the biceps tendon.

Look for a thin soft spot in the tendon at the point of maximal pain. This is the site of the strain. With tendinitis there can be tendon thickening with stiffness and pain.

Assessment: Pain will decrease and active range of motion will increase.

Light Treatment Plan: In mild to moderate cases, a total average dose of 25–600 joules can be administered to the attachment points of the tendon plus an equal amount of joules for painting the surrounding area. This may stimulate healing, while reducing swelling and pain; it also can be useful in reducing any scarring from surgery. Treat every two or three days until recovery is evident.

Adjunctive Treatment Plan: Prescribe gentle muscle strengthening and stretching once healing has occurred sufficiently to allow the tissues to accept stress. For tendinitis, friction massage may help. Taping can be used during the acute stage of a strain to prevent further tearing and assist in rehabilitation. It can be helpful to alternate ice and heat to control inflammation and pain. If the problem persists after appropriate therapy, consider a referral to an orthopedic specialist.

Carpal Tunnel Syndrome

(diagram page 84, dose page 82)

Subjective: Symptoms are numbness and/or pain in the thumb and/or middle three fingers that can increase with activity or at night while sleeping. In moderate to severe cases the pain can be disabling and radiate up into the forearm and arm.

Assessment: Successful treatment results produce decreased pain and increased function and strength.

Light Treatment Plan: The light must be aimed at the median nerve in the carpal tunnel both vertically and slightly angled to either side of the tendons in the wrist to bathe the entire nerve in photons. A treatment dose of approximately 25 to 100 joules is initially administered in most cases, less if the pain is acute or severe.

It may also be advisable to treat the adjacent tender points in the forearm and hand with 5 to 25 joules per point or perform nerve tracing over the median nerve into the hand. Fingernails can be painted with 10 to 50 joules if additional peripheral stimulation is needed. Always consider the possibility of treating the brachial nerves in the lateral/anterior neck or at the spinal level if you believe that the problem could be cervicogenic.

Treatment can start daily for up to three or four days or until symptoms decrease. Chronic conditions may require higher doses up to 300 joules with a high power laser and frequency can be two or three times a week for up to four weeks.

Adjunctive Treatment Plan: Daily, gentle flexion and extension stretching of the wrist can be added as long as it does not aggravate symptoms. It can be helpful to initially use ice and then alternate ice and heat directly over the carpal tunnel to control inflammation and pain. Many patients find benefit from bracing, especially at night. If the problem persists after appropriate therapy, consider a referral to an orthopedic specialist for injections or surgical intervention.

Fractured Finger or Wrist

(diagram page 84, dose page 82)

Subjective: Pain can be mild to severe at the fracture site. The patient may have already been treated by an orthopedic specialist and received x-rays, fracture reduction, casting, and possibly surgery.

Assessment: Decreased pain and swelling with increased range of motion.

Light Treatment Plan: Acute conditions can be treated immediately to reduce swelling and pain with about 25 to 200 joules at the site fracture and the surrounding strained soft tissues. If a cast is in place, treatment can be applied to the arteries above the fracture site with 25 to 200 joules per treatment to stimulate healing in the forearm region. You may also treat the radial or ulnar arteries if the cast is on the hand. Once the temporary or plaster cast has been removed, light treatments may resume two or more times per week until an acceptable level of healing has occurred.

Adjunctive Treatment Plan: In cases of non-union, bone healing may be aided with light therapy. Be certain that the patient eats a balanced diet and consider multi-mineral supplementation. It can be helpful to alternate ice/heat to stimulate circulation and control inflammation and pain once the cast has been removed. In many cases, there will be decreased range of motion that will require gentle active followed by passive range of motion activities. If the problem persists after appropriate therapy, consider referral to an orthopedic specialist for further evaluation.

Fractured Clavicle (diagram page 85, dose page 82)

Subjective: Mild to severe pain at the fracture site.

Assessment: Decreased pain and swelling indicate improvement.

Light Treatment Plan: The majority of fractures are in acute or sub-acute conditions and light can be applied even before x-rays and a sling have been provided to speed healing and reduce swelling and pain. An average treatment dose of 25 to 200 joules is applied directly over and around the fracture site. Treatment can also be initiated soon after diagnosis and treatment by a physician have been completed and the fracture has been stabilized. After the bone has been reset, treatment can be administered every two to three days until pain and swelling have been reduced.

Adjunctive Treatment Plan: In cases of non-union fractures, light therapy may improve bone healing. Patients should eat a balanced diet and consider multi-mineral supplementation. It can be helpful to initially use ice and later alternate ice/heat to control inflammation and pain. If the problem persists after appropriate therapy, consider a referral back to the orthopedic specialist.

Frozen Shoulder (diagram page 85, dose page 82)

Subjective: Stiffness and pain in and around the shoulder joint, difficulty sleeping, and pain with motion, especially abduction.

Assessment: Improved active and passive range of motion; lessened pain.

Light Treatment Plan: Acute conditions can be treated with a total dose of 50 to 600 joules. This can be administered at approximately 10 to 25 joules to various points, directed to the center of the shoulder joint from the anterior, posterior, and superior aspects. The surrounding area may also be painted with approximately 25 to 100 joules. Treatment can be done every two or three days until the patient has achieved 90% of normal range of motion.

Adjunctive Treatment Plan: Passive and active mobilization is a vital part of the therapy. Passive mobilization can be performed in all appropriate directions including posterior, inferior, and lateral glide as well as abduction and adduction. Gentle stretching at home, two to three times per day, is important. It can be helpful to alternate ice and heat to control inflammation and pain. In some cases acupuncture and taping can provide benefit. If the problem persists after appropriate therapy, consider a referral to an orthopedic specialist for manipulation under anesthesia.

Rotator Cuff Strain

(diagram page 83, dose page 82)

Subjective: Pain is usually felt with abduction. If rupture is moderate or severe, pain can also be present at rest, with swelling, bruising, and muscle weakness.

Assessment: Active range of motion will gradually become more pain-free.

Light Treatment Plan: Acute conditions can be treated with an average dose of 25 to 200 joules applied to the injured area with a combination of point treatment and painting. Treatments should be given every two to three days until satisfactory relief is achieved.

Adjunctive Treatment Plan: Gentle strengthening when there is no pain associated with effort. Taping can help stabilize the muscle during the acute stage. Alternating ice and heat may control inflammation and pain. If the problem persists after appropriate therapy, consider a referral to an orthopedic specialist.

Tennis and Golfer's Elbow

(diagram page 85, dose page 82)

Subjective: This is also called lateral or medial epicondylitis. Pain is present on palpation at the medial or lateral epicondyle tendon attachment sites. Although the problem can occur from participation in sports, almost any repetitive forearm and hand activity can create this condition. Patients may report difficulty lifting a coffee cup or carton of milk, shaking hands, or opening doors.

Assessment: With increasing healing, there will be less pain, increased ability to lift heavier objects with the hand, and improved functional activities.

Light Treatment Plan: This condition can be treated with a total average dose of 20 to 100 joules. This dose can be administered to tender points adjacent to the epicondyles as well as directly on the attachment site for 5 to 50 joules per point, followed by painting over the region near the epicondyle. Treatments can be done two to three times a week for two to six weeks, with decreasing frequency as symptoms abate.

Adjunctive Treatment Plan: In acute cases ice and heat can assist in symptom control. In chronic cases, friction, trigger point or myofascial massage, spray/stretch, and gentle strengthening can be beneficial when appropriate. No massage on the epicondyle is recommended in the acute stage, and stretching should start only after the pain has significantly decreased. Using a tennis elbow brace and taping during upper-extremity activities can be protective.

Thumb or Finger Sprain

(diagram page 86, dose page 82)

Subjective: Pain with active and/or passive range of motion.

Assessment: There will be decreasing subjective complaints and improved range of motion and strength.

Light Treatment Plan: Treatment can be given two to five times the first week and directed into the joint space from all four sides .

Adjunctive Treatment Plan: Gentle, active range of motion may be indicated in the first week if it causes no aggravation of symptoms. Passive range of motion or mobilization can be performed once the acute injury has stabilized. It can be helpful to initially use ice and then ice/heat to control inflammation and pain. Bracing and taping can reduce pain and prevent further injury. If the problem persists after appropriate therapy, consider a referral to an orthopedic specialist.

Arm or Forearm Tendinitis

(diagram page 86, dose page 82)

Subjective: The patient will notice loss of function due to forearm pain.

Assessment: Improvement will be noted as decreased pain, increased strength, and improved function.

Light Treatment Plan: This condition can be treated with a total average treatment dose of approximately 50 to 600 joules. This dose can be administered to tender points, followed by painting.

Remember that deeper points require longer treatment times. Treatment can be given once or twice a week for two to six weeks or until relief is obtained.

Adjunctive Treatment Plan: In acute cases initially using ice and then ice/heat can assist in symptom control. In chronic and subacute cases, friction, trigger point or myofascial massage, spray/stretch, home application of ice or heat, and stretching can be beneficial. Night bracing is often protective.

Upper Body Diagrams

Typical Treatment Time and Joules based on Power of Device

Probe Output (mW)	Joules	Treatment Time
10	6 - 12	10 - 20 mins
100	36 - 72	6 - 12 mins
500	60 - 180	2 - 6 mins
1,000	90 - 240	1.5 - 4 mins
2,000	120 - 360	1 - 3 mins
4,000	240 - 480	1 - 2 mins
6,000	270 - 540	.75 - 1.5 mins
8,000	240 - 600	.5 - 1.25 mins
10,000	150 - 600	.25 - 1 min

The above chart notes the approximate treatment times based on the power of the device being used. Since the suggested treatment doses in this book are for LEDs in the range of 10 to 10,000 mW, full body treatment times will be approximately 1–15 minutes and approximately 100 to 1200 joules. If you are using a lower power LED, you will need to use longer treatment times, and proportionally less joules.

Use this chart as a guide for an approximate treatment time and dosage based on your particular LED and the individual needs of the patient.

Upper Body

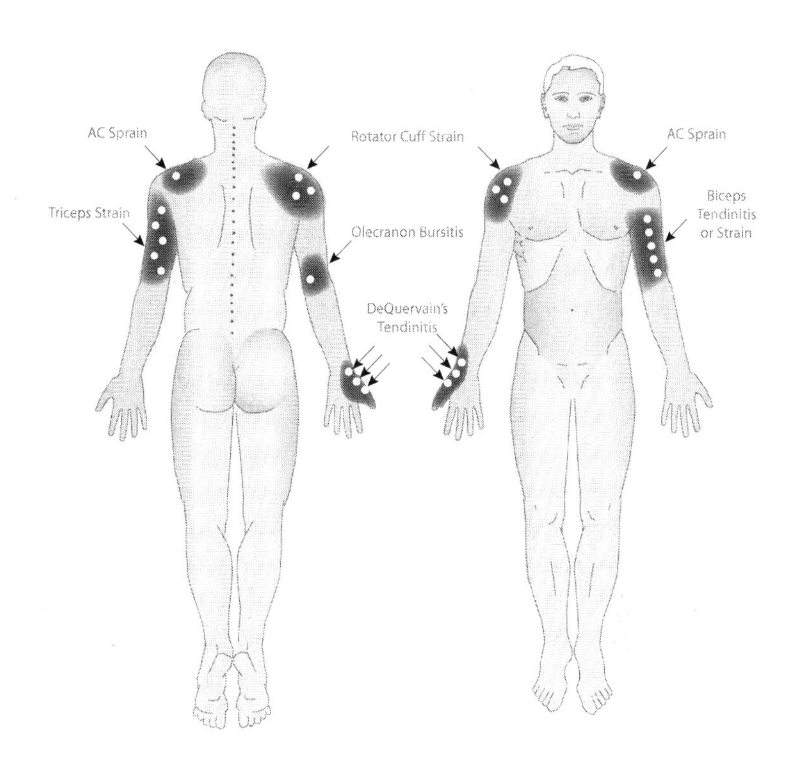
AC Sprain
Rotator Cuff Strain
AC Sprain
Triceps Strain
Biceps
Tendinitis
or Strain
Olecranon Bursitis
DeQuervain's
Tendinitis

Upper Body

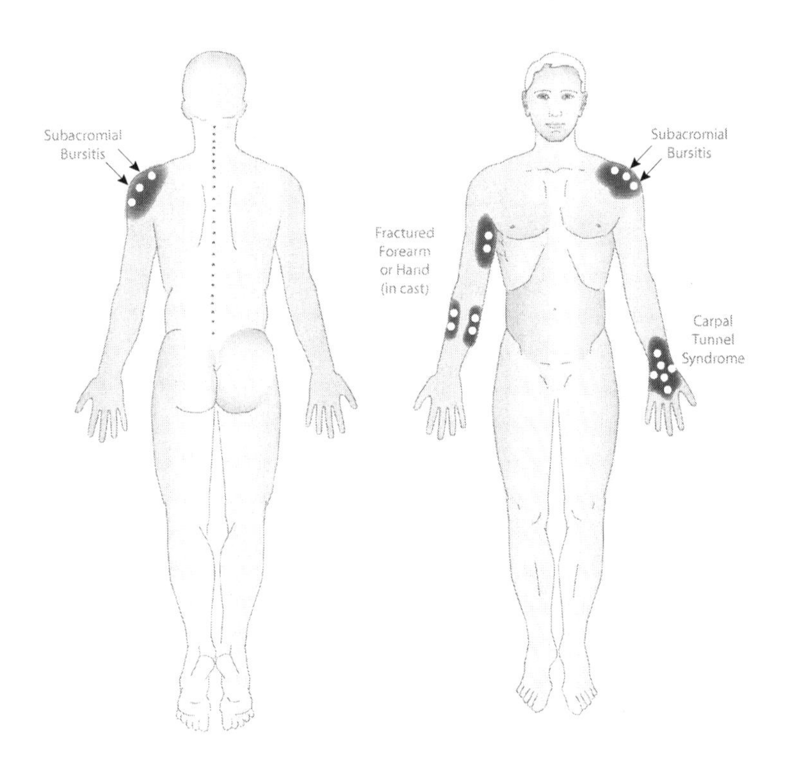
Subacromial
Bursitis
Subacromial
Bursitis
Fractured
Forearm
or Hand
(in cast)
Carpal
Tunnel
Syndrome

Upper Body

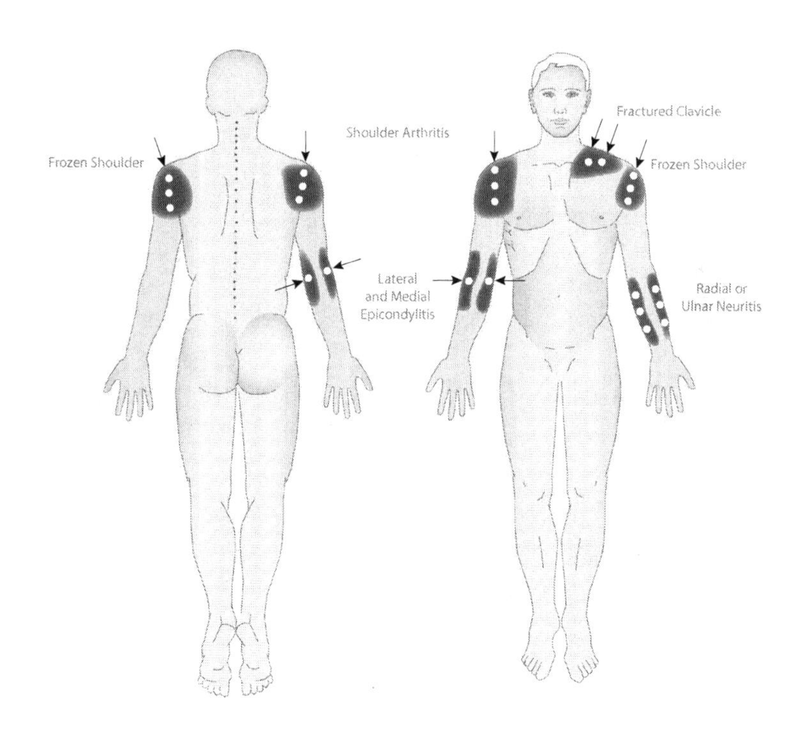
Frozen Shoulder
Shoulder Arthritis
Fractured Clavicle
Frozen Shoulder
Lateral
and Medial
Epicondylitis
Radial or
Ulnar Neuritis

Upper Body

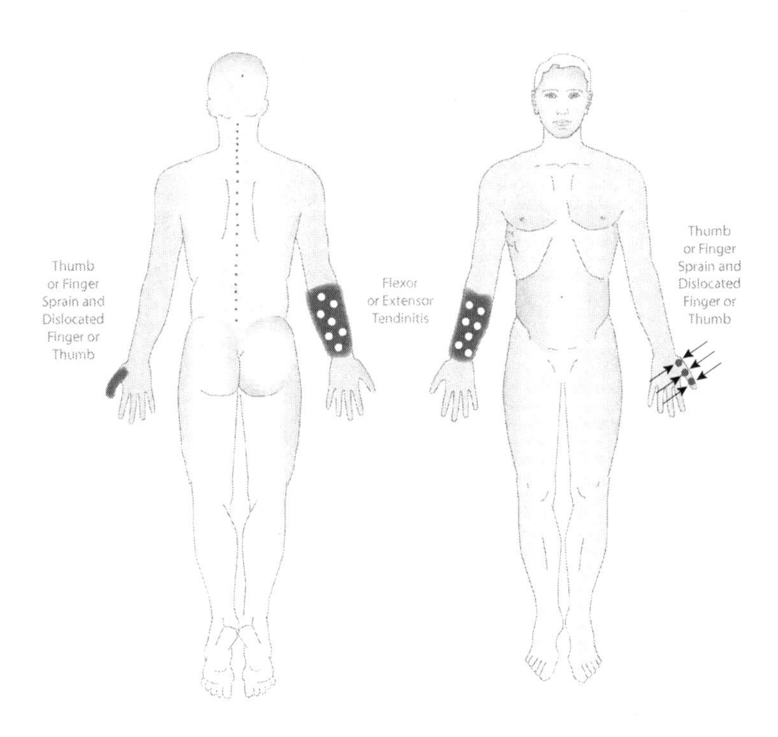
Thumb
or Finger
Sprain and
Dislocated
Finger or
Thumb
Flexor
or Extensor
Tendinitis
Thumb
or Finger
Sprain and
Dislocated
Finger or
Thumb

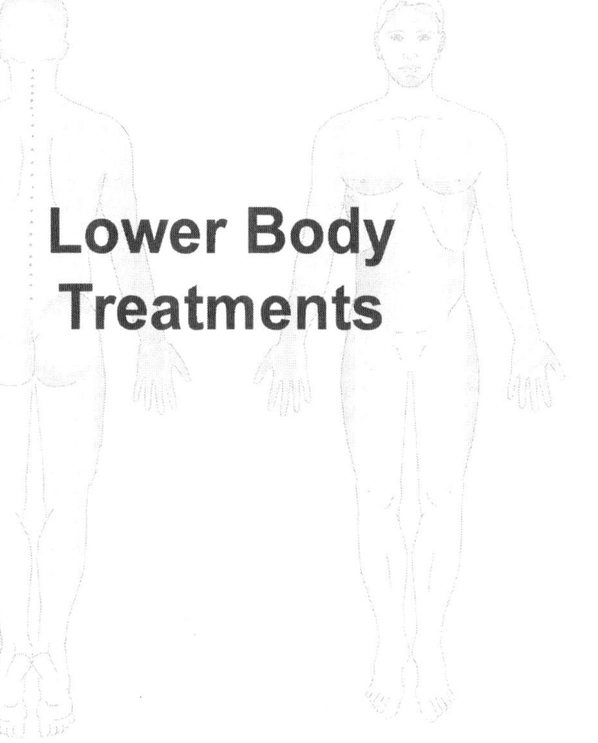

Lower Body Treatments

Achilles Tendinitis

(diagram page 104, dose page 102)

Subjective: The patient will complain of heel pain or pain in the lower calf. The problem is common in track and field sports, dancers, and not uncommon in the majority of sports.

Assessment: There will be improved ability to do pain-free, standing toe raises.

Light Treatment Plan: Acute conditions can be treated with a total dose of 50 to 600 joules, with the primary focus being the site of the tendon strain, followed by painting over the general area. Treatment can be given every two to three days, decreasing treatment frequency as the condition heals. Direct the photons from posterior to anterior as well as from a lateral and medial position and at an anterior angle to the tendon to infiltrate its frontal aspect. If the patient has been treated surgically, treat in a similar manner as soon as possible, even daily, until swelling and pain have decreased.

Adjunctive Treatment Plan: When the tendon has healed and the patient can walk pain-free, then gentle stretching of the calf but not the tendon should begin. Wearing heel lifts or high heels can reduce strain on an injured Achilles tendon. Reserve stretching of the tendon and gentle strengthening until the Achilles has fully healed and exercise can be performed without pain. Taping of the tendon can help stabilize the weakened tissue.

Anterior and Posterior Cruciate Ligament Injury

(diagram page 106, dose page 102)

Subjective: The patient often complains of a knee "popping," "giving out" or becoming weak. There may be reports of a "click" or a straining sensation in the knee while playing sports that require "cutting" or jumping. The patient may be limping and usually complains that the knee is painful, stiff, and swollen. The severity of the subjective complaints is usually proportional to the degree of ligament strain or rupture.

Assessment: Improvement will show as decreased pain and swelling, with improved range of motion. In milder cases, as symptoms improve, there will be less instability with the Lachman and Drawer tests.

Light Treatment Plan: Acute conditions can be treated with a dose of 25 to 300 joules. Only titrate if improvement is evident with a slow increase in dose. The treatment can be divided into four to five entry points on the knee joint, directed along the joint line, at the posterior, medial and lateral aspects of the knee as well as lateral and medial to the patella. Keep the light in one position, if possible, at each point, to increase depth of penetration. Add painting over the knee if pain covers a broad area, or if using a high power device. Treatment can be given daily for up to five days, followed by decreasing frequency as long as progress is maintained.

Adjunctive Treatment Plan: If the knee cannot be flexed or extended, the condition should be assessed by an orthopedic specialist. Straight leg-raising exercises, with the knee in a gently extended position, and, when pain free, gentle use of the stationary bike, can be used to tone the quadriceps. Begin additional strength training as soon as possible, teaching the patient unloaded, isometric strengthening exercises before progressing to loading and bending the knee. Strength and agility must be attained before the patient can engage in more vigorous activities. Ice/heat, taping or a knee brace can support the injury during the acute stage. Serious ruptures usually need to be surgically repaired.

Calf Strain (diagram page 105, dose page 102)

Subjective: There is pain in the gastrocnemius or soleus muscles usually brought on by explosive exercise or excessive stretching. The patient, in moderate cases, may exhibit a limp and have difficulty dorsiflexing the ankle due to spasm.

Assessment: There will be a return to pain-free range of motion and normal strength in plantar flexion.

Light Treatment Plan: An acute calf strain can be treated with a treatment dose of approximately 50 to 600 joules. This can be administered to tender points of about 10 to 25 joules over the most painful points, followed by painting over a larger muscle area. Usually this problem is self-limiting and treatment two to three times per week for one to two weeks will be sufficient. If the strain looks severe, be certain that an Achilles tendon tear is not present.

Adjunctive Treatment Plan: Begin self-help passive stretching as soon as it is comfortable. Do not encourage vigorous activity until the muscle has healed well.

Hamstring Strain and Tendinitis

(diagram page 103, dose page 102)

Subjective: There is tenderness of the proximal or distal insertion of one of the hamstring muscles of the posterior thigh. If it is a muscle strain, the pain will be more toward the middle of the posterior thigh.

Assessment: With improvement there will be decreased tenderness on palpation and increasingly pain-free activity.

Light Treatment Plan: The hamstring bursa or tendon can be treated with a dose of about 25 to 200 joules. Following this, tender points can be treated or the area can be painted with approximately 10 to 50 joules. The pain is often significantly reduced after two to five treatments in the acute stage, slightly more with chronic conditions.

Adjunctive Treatment Plan: Stretching the hamstring with the leg slightly adducted or abducted, depending on the muscle involved, can improve flexibility in the medial and lateral compartments. Use of ice/heat for five minutes, five times per day can help in the acute stage of injury.

Hip Sprain (diagram page 104, dose page 102)

Subjective: Pain will be felt in the middle of the groin and may radiate to the thigh or knee. In many ways, this condition may resemble a pubic sprain, groin strain, or hip arthritis. However, unlike with arthritis, there may be an acute incident, involving extreme hip extension or flexion precipitating this injury. Note also that hip arthritis rarely occurs in patients under 50 years old.

Assessment: Treatment will create a rapid decrease in symptoms.

Light Treatment Plan: Treat with 50 to 600 joules directly over the anterior acetabulum. Posterior treatment of the acetabulum can be accomplished by treating the sciatic notch and aiming the photon stream toward the hip socket. Treatment two times per week for one to two weeks is often sufficient for a mild to moderate injury.

Adjunctive Treatment Plan: Gentle active range of motion can be encouraged but extreme passive or active range of motion should not be performed until the joint has fully healed. Strengthening of the hip muscles is imperative.

Metatarsalgia—Morton's Neuroma

(diagram page 105, dose page 102)

Subjective: Many patients present with an intermittent dull ache, cramping, numbness or burning, and occasional shooting pain in the plantar aspects of the metatarsal interspaces. Symptoms usually worsen with weight-bearing activity and improve with rest.

In chronic cases of Morton's Neuroma, a lump of scar tissue will form and there is a palpable mass under the ball of the foot, which will be painful when weight is applied to the metatarsal heads. Pain can also be increased on palpation over the metatarsal heads or with range of motion.

Assessment: With treatment, there will be decreased pain, numbness, and cramping, and improved functional activities.

Light Treatment Plan: Acute and chronic conditions can be treated with a dose of 50 to 300 joules. This can be directed at the interdigital nerves between the metatarsal heads.

Adjunctive Treatment Plan: It can be helpful to alternate ice/heat to control inflammation and pain. Referral to a podiatrist or orthopedic doctor for orthotics, injections, or surgery may also be necessary if there is no improvement.

Knee Meniscus or Ligament Sprain/Strain

(diagram page 104, dose page 102)

Subjective: The patient will complain of pain deep inside the knee and often recall an instance of a feeling that something snapped or strained.

Objective: When the medial and/or lateral knee joint becomes inflamed due to strain or tearing, the knee will swell within the first few hours thereafter and can stay swollen for days to weeks, depending on the severity of the strain. The knee may also feel weak, like it is going to buckle, or lock into one position. An MRI will usually improve the accuracy of this diagnosis. Always test for damage to the anterior and posterior cruciate ligaments as the two syndromes can occur simultaneously.

Assessment: There will be less swelling and increasingly pain-free range of motion with an improved sense of stability and strength.

Light Treatment Plan: Acute conditions can be treated with a dose of 25 to 100 joules. In some cases up to 600 joules per session will be needed. Only increase the dosage if condition shows improvement with each gentle titration. This can be directed to the medial and lateral joint line, the posterior knee, and points just lateral and medical to the patella. Keep the light in one position in each point, if possible, to increase depth of penetration. Add painting all over the knee if swelling is present. Treatment can be given daily for up to five days, decreasing frequency as long as progress is maintained.

Adjunctive Treatment Plan: If the knee cannot be flexed or extended, an orthopedic specialist should assess the patient immediately. Institute straight leg raising exercises with the knee in a gently extended position, and do not add knee flexion until it is comfortably tolerated and only in the subacute phase. Taping is important to stabilize the joint. Once the knee is stable, very gentle joint mobilization may improve mobility if there is reduced range of motion.

Kneecap and Quadriceps Tendinitis

(diagrams pages 103 & 105, dose page 102)

Subjective: This strain involves the quadriceps muscles and often includes the rectus femoris, vastus lateralis, vastus medialis, and the vastus intermedius. This muscle group becomes inflamed at their insertion on the superior or inferior patellar regions. Pain can be felt when the superior or inferior end of the patella is touched, walking up and down stairs, or performing any repeated knee flexion and extension. There may also be redness and swelling in the area.

Assessment: There will be decreasing pain and swelling and increased ability to engage in functional and athletic activities.

Light Treatment Plan: Treat with 25 to 200 joules directly over the inflamed tendon/ligament, angling the probe posteriorly, medially and laterally to bathe all sides of the knee in photons. Treatment is usually effective when provided one to two times per week; more frequent sessions can be helpful in the most severe cases. Often two to ten treatments are necessary depending on the chronicity of the condition.

Adjunctive Treatment Plan: Hip extension stretching can be helpful, if appropriate, adding strengthening exercises as rehabilitation progresses. It can be helpful to use alternate ice/heat to control inflammation and pain. If the problem persists after appropriate therapy, consider a referral to an orthopedic specialist.

Peripheral Neuropathy (PN)

(diagram page 104, dose page 102)

Subjective: Symptoms may include numbness, loss of balance, burning, tightness, hypersensitivity to touch, and motor weakness in the feet and/or legs.

Assessment: A small percentage of patients will achieve complete remission after 4 to 12 sessions, but most will get temporary relief for 1 to 5 days.

Light Treatment Plan: Start with 10–100 joules per foot and increase dosage if treatment is well tolerated. PN is difficult to treat because some patients become more symptomatic after 25 joules of treatment and others feel relief when they receive more than 500 J per foot, for a total of more than 1,000 J! Spend 2/3 of the time treating the most symptomatic points on the bottom of the foot, followed by painting. Spend 1/3 of the time treating the top of the foot or the popliteal fossa to stimulate the popliteal artery.

Adjunctive Treatment Plan: In general, optimal weight, a regular exercise program, a balanced diet, nutritional supplements, and limiting alcohol consumption can reduce symptoms. Some physicians have found that topical and oral L-Arginine can be of benefit. Nutritional support often involves a multivitamin and mineral formula with Alpha Lipoic Acid, L-carnitine, Benfotiamine, B vitamins, and other nutrients.

Plantar Fasciitis (diagram page 103, dose page 102)

Subjective: The typical pain pattern is sharp pain along the middle to posterior arch of the sole of the foot. It may occasionally occur with a heel spur. Patients complain of plantar pain, particularly with the first few steps in the morning or after periods of inactivity. Excessive weight, pregnancy, repeated damage from jumping and other high impact activities, and flat feet can be causative.

Assessment: Treatment often results in a slow, steady decrease in pain and improved ability to engage in impact activity.

Light Treatment Plan: Start with 25–100 joules and titrate up slowly if there is an improvement in symptoms after each session. Half of the treatment should be focused on the painful points in the plantar fascia with the other half of the joules utilized painting over the symptomatic area. Begin treating three times per week and decrease frequency as symptoms improve.

Adjunctive Treatment Plan: During the acute phase, the patient should use ice or ice/heat on a regular basis. Taping and orthotics can be helpful. The patient should focus on non-weight bearing activities such as swimming and bicycling. In the subacute phase, regular stretching of the sole of the foot and Achilles can be valuable. As the plantar fascia heals and to reduce scar tissue, massage of the plantar fascia, can be quite helpful. If conservative therapy is not successful, referral to a podiatrist or orthopedic specialist is necessary.

Restless Leg Syndrome or Leg Cramps

(diagram page 103, dose page 102)

Subjective: Patients complain of involuntary sudden movement of the legs. In many cases patients may be unaware of having Restless Leg Syndrome (RLS) until it is brought to their attention when they kick a companion while sleeping. Leg cramps are also usually present.

Assessment: Patients will report a decrease of involuntary kicks while sleeping and/or have fewer cramps.

Light Treatment Plan: Treat trigger, tender or acupuncture points in the low back, hip, and lower extremity with 10 to 25 joules per point. Treatment can be applied two times per week for two to three weeks.

Adjunctive Treatment Plan: Regular gentle leg and foreleg/calf stretching is vital. Sometimes stretching after heat can improve the effectiveness of the stretching. Make sure the patient has good nutrition and proper intake of minerals.

Shin Splints (diagram page 105, dose page 102)

Subjective: The patient complains of pain along the medial aspect of the tibialis anterior and, in many cases, along the anterolateral tibia, usually following an increase in jogging or hiking prior to onset of symptoms.

Assessment: Pain-free walking and then jogging is a sign of tissue healing.

Light Treatment Plan: Acute conditions of shin splints can be treated with a total average treatment dose of 25 to 200 joules. This can be administered to tender points with 10 to 25 joules per point followed by painting the surrounding area.

Adjunctive Treatment Plan: Make sure that the patient has good lower extremity biomechanics and good athletic shoes. Begin gentle strength training to the anterior compartment muscles as soon as it is comfortable and add stretching and massage once the tissue is in the subacute stage.

Sprained Ankle (diagram page 105, dose page 102)

Subjective: Ankle pain with stiffness.

Assessment: There will be increased range of motion, less pain, and decreased swelling.

Light Treatment Plan: A sprained ankle can be treated with a total average dose of 50 to 300 joules. This can be administered to the local area of the sprain with approximately 5 to 15 joules per point, especially on the lateral aspect, followed by painting over the whole ankle. Treatment can be given every two to three days for one to three weeks or until the condition is healed.

Adjunctive Treatment Plan: A strength and conditioning program can be helpful. Encourage the patient to warm up before practice or competition and use tape to stabilize the ankle. It may be important to use an ankle brace and supportive shoes in some cases. If the condition becomes chronic or the patient is a competitive athlete, use of a balance board and other ankle exercises to increase strength, balance, and proprioception may be indicated.

Tensor Fascia Lata and Iliotibial Band Syndrome (diagram page 104, dose page 102)

Subjective: The patient complains of pain above or below the greater trochanter. It may present as a point of pain or mimic sciatica and radiate from the lateral buttock into the lateral knee. This is a common problem in runners and other athletes, but can also be associated with an earlier bout of sciatica or in out-of-shape patients who do not engage in regular stretching.

Assessment: Treatment should result in less pain on palpation, increased flexibility, improved range of motion, and a return to pain-free activity.

Light Treatment Plan: Acute conditions can be treated with a dose of 25 to 50 joules. In some cases, if the patient tolerates the treatment well, increasing to 100–300 joules may be indicated if both conditions are present. Treatment can be administered above and below the greater trochanter and distally to the lateral condyle of the tibia. Treat each tender point with 5 to 25 joules and then paint over the entire symptomatic area.

Adjunctive Treatment Plan: When treating athletes, it may be important to encourage them to have a coach assess their athletic form or have a foot specialist watch their gait and lower extremity biomechanics. Myofascial or trigger point massage, self-massage with a foam roll, and spray/stretch may be added to reduce spasm and fibrous adhesions. It can be helpful to institute active stretching of abductors, within a pain-free range, once the patient's symptoms have stabilized. Reduce activity to a level that does not generate pain and try applying ice/heat to the region of pain along the ITB or TFL to control symptoms.

Tibial or Fibula Stress Fracture

(diagram page 105, dose page 102)

Subjective: The patient complains of pain along the shaft of the tibia or fibula.

Assessment: There will be pain-free walking, running, and stretching.

Light Treatment Plan: Acute conditions can be treated with approximately 25 to 200 joules. This can be administered at about 25–50 joules per point along the painful aspect of the tibia or fibula. Treatment can be given every one to two days until improvement is evident.

Adjunctive Treatment Plan: Often gentle weight bearing and later strength training will help stimulate healing. Avoiding anything that aggravates the pain is very important.

Lower Body Diagrams

Typical Treatment Time and Joules based on Power of Device

Probe Output (mW)	Joules	Treatment Time
10	6 - 12	10 - 20 mins
100	36 - 72	6 - 12 mins
500	60 - 180	2 - 6 mins
1,000	90 - 240	1.5 - 4 mins
2,000	120 - 360	1 - 3 mins
4,000	240 - 480	1 - 2 mins
6,000	270 - 540	.75 - 1.5 mins
8,000	240 - 600	.5 - 1.25 mins
10,000	150 - 600	.25 - 1 min

The above chart notes the approximate treatment times based on the power of the device being used. Since the suggested treatment doses in this book are for LEDs in the range of 10 to 10,000 mW, full body treatment times will be approximately 1–15 minutes and approximately 100 to 1200 joules. If you are using a lower power LED, you will need to use longer treatment times, and proportionally less joules.

Use this chart as a guide for an approximate treatment time and dosage based on your particular LED and the individual needs of the patient.

Lower Body

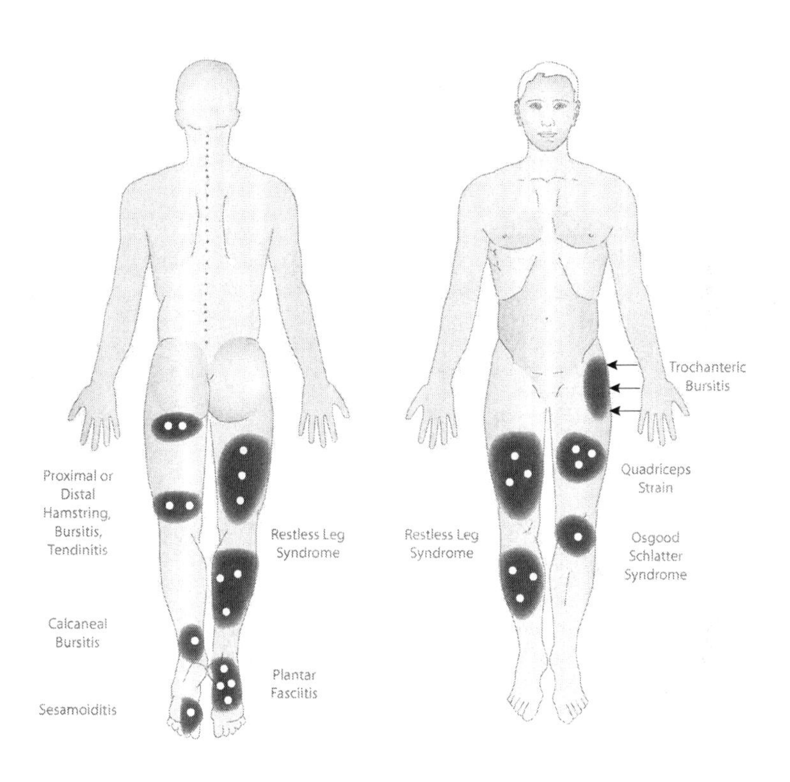
Proximal or
Distal
Hamstring,
Bursitis,
Tendinitis
Calcaneal
Bursitis
Sesamoiditis
Restless Leg
Syndrome
Plantar
Fasciitis
Restless Leg
Syndrome
Trochanteric
Bursitis
Quadriceps
Strain
Osgood
Schlatter
Syndrome

Lower Body

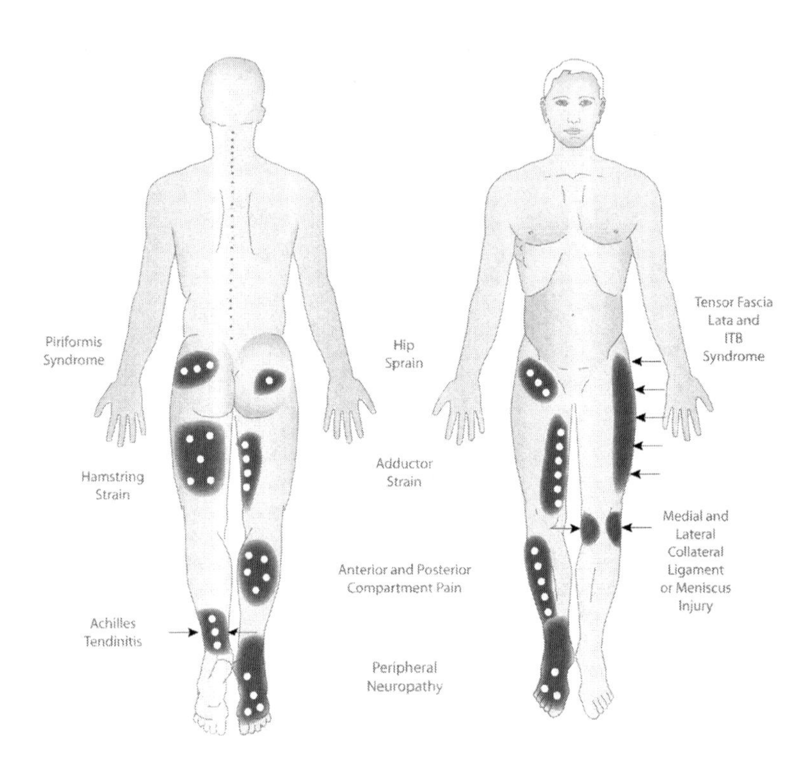
Piriformis Syndrome
Hip Sprain
Tensor Fascia Lata and ITB Syndrome
Hamstring Strain
Adductor Strain
Medial and Lateral Collateral Ligament or Meniscus Injury
Anterior and Posterior Compartment Pain
Achilles Tendinitis
Peripheral Neuropathy

Lower Body

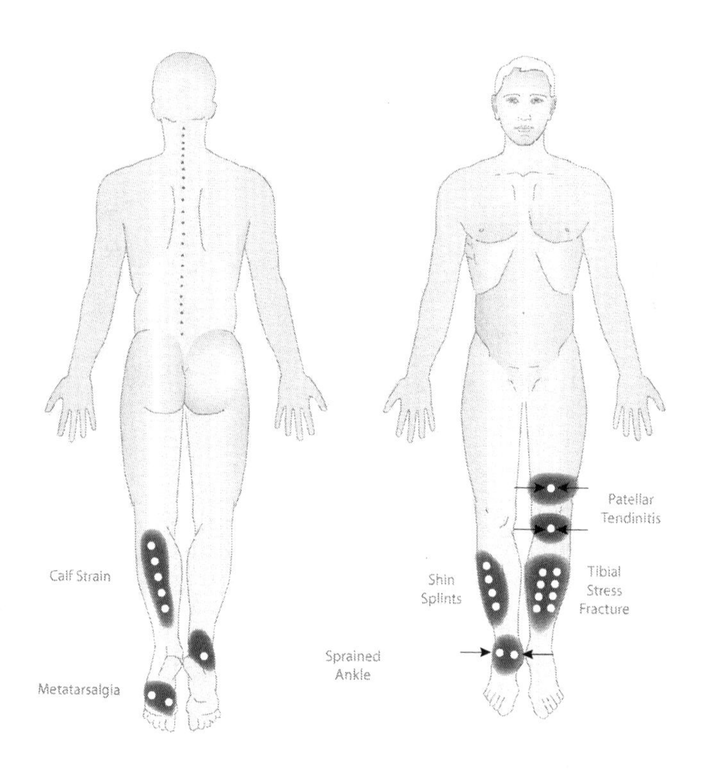
Calf Strain
Metatarsalgia
Sprained Ankle
Patellar Tendinitis
Shin Splints
Tibial Stress Fracture

Lower Body

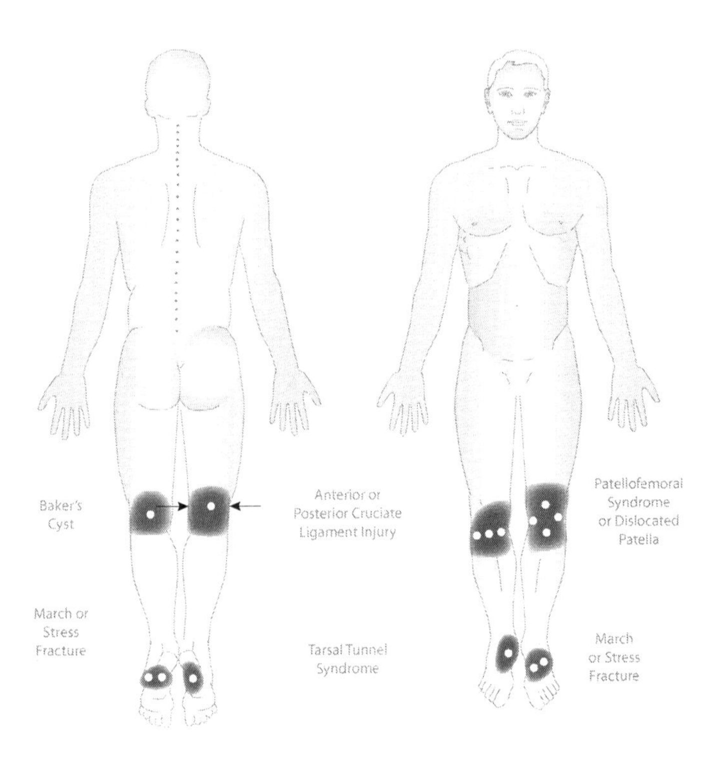
Baker's
Cyst
Anterior or
Posterior Cruciate
Ligament Injury
Patellofemoral
Syndrome
or Dislocated
Patella
March or
Stress
Fracture
Tarsal Tunnel
Syndrome
March
or Stress
Fracture

Brain Treatments

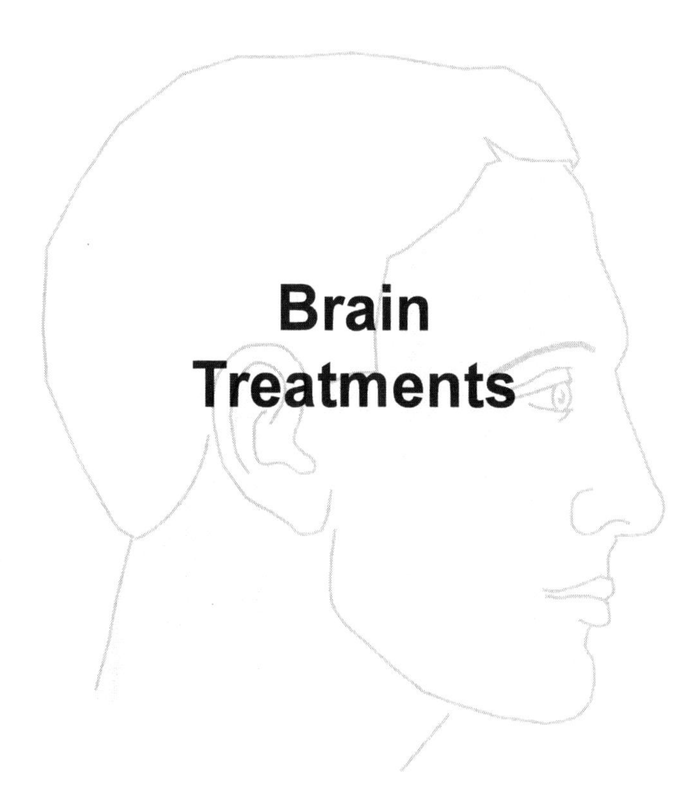

Treating the Brain (diagram page 115)

One of the most exciting discoveries in light and laser science has been proof that light can improve healing of the brain. Even though studies began in 2005 on animals and many have been performed more recently on humans, the FDA has not looked at these treatments sufficiently to warrant FDA clearance. However, the compelling data from this research warrants inclusion into any book on light therapy. I will present some basic protocols for treating the brain based on the latest research. If you are interested in learning more, there are many excellent studies coming out of the Wellman Centers for Photomedicine at Harvard Medical School and Massachusetts General Hospital, as well as many studies from Europe, Asia, and the Middle East.

Be careful

Please exercise caution, as this information is taken from the research literature and is not an FDA-cleared indication for using LEDs. We legally cannot treat the brain. However, remember that whenever you treat the head for headaches or muscular head pain (like the temporalis muscle), you are also treating the brain! The same thing occurs when you treat over the spine for back pain. You are, in fact, treating the spinal cord as well!

Benefits have been proven

We are not sure exactly how light therapy improves brain function, but we do know that it has many positive effects that can last for weeks or months after treatment. These long-term changes must be due to a significant improvement with brain physiology and function. Some researchers believe it is due to improved ATP synthesis, increased blood flow, or improved oxygenation, even though these probably do not explain all of the long-term improvements that have been noted with traumatic brain injury, stroke, and Alzheimer's/dementia.

Wavelength

As mentioned in other parts of this book, we do know that there are some wavelengths that are more effective than others. We know that 660 nm and 810 nm are often considered the most effective wavelengths for many types of light and laser therapy because these wavelengths are powerfully absorbed. In general, 810 nm produces the most effective penetration and is the most thoroughly studied. Studies show that higher wavelenths produce very deep penetration as well. These longer wavelengths above 1,000 nm can be effective, but because they generate more heat, especially with higher power lasers, they tend to be avoided in brain research.

LED vs. Laser

We are now seeing an increase in the use of LEDs rather than lasers in brain research and for other types of light and laser therapy because they are less expensive and quite effective. This may make them more useful than lasers when treating the brain, unless the laser has a low total output power and power density, to ensure that it is cool and safe. For example, a high-powered, collimated 10,000 mW hot laser has risks when treating the brain that do not occur with a lower power laser or an LED.

Dosage

Dosage is a controversial subject when treating spine and extremity injuries, but it becomes more complex when treating the brain. In summary, it has been shown that, in the human skull, penetration could reach approximately 1–2 inches (40–50 mm). Whether you are treating animals or humans, it has also been shown that earlier intervention and repeated treatments are the most effective way to produce long-lasting results. From what we see in the literature, one treatment to an area of old brain trauma will be unlikely to produce any significant benefit.

Here is a typical treatment protocol:

Let's invent a study that uses a 500 mW LED that is applied to each side of the forehead for 4 minutes. If you have a 3,000 mW device, you would reduce the time proportionally:

1. So, 4 minutes (240 seconds) divided by 6 equals 40 seconds. Because a 3,000 mW device is 6 times stronger than a 500 mW device, you would reduce the dose to 1/6 of the dose compared to a lower power light device.
2. Thus, you could gently paint over each side of the prefrontal cortex for 40 seconds.
3. Note: Since a 3,000 mW device produces 180 joules per minute and you treat both sides of the forehead for 30 seconds, your total dose would be about 180 joules. However, remember that only a small percentage of those joules reach the brain!

Where Do You Treat?

Most of the studies treating emotional and cognitive function treat the prefrontal cortex. However, a study of Parkinson's disease applied light to the brain stem, as well as the occipital, parietal, temporal, and frontal lobes, and along the sagittal suture. Treating the sagittal suture, because it is just superior to the saggital sinus, could be an excellent area of treatment to improve blood and CSF flow. Remember that studies show that light has systemic effects, so you can treat almost anywhere in the body, even the feet, and have a mild effect on the brain!

If you are interested in learning how the researchers decidced what areas to treat, just do an Internet search on "Brain Function Map" and you will find lots of resources to help guide your studies.

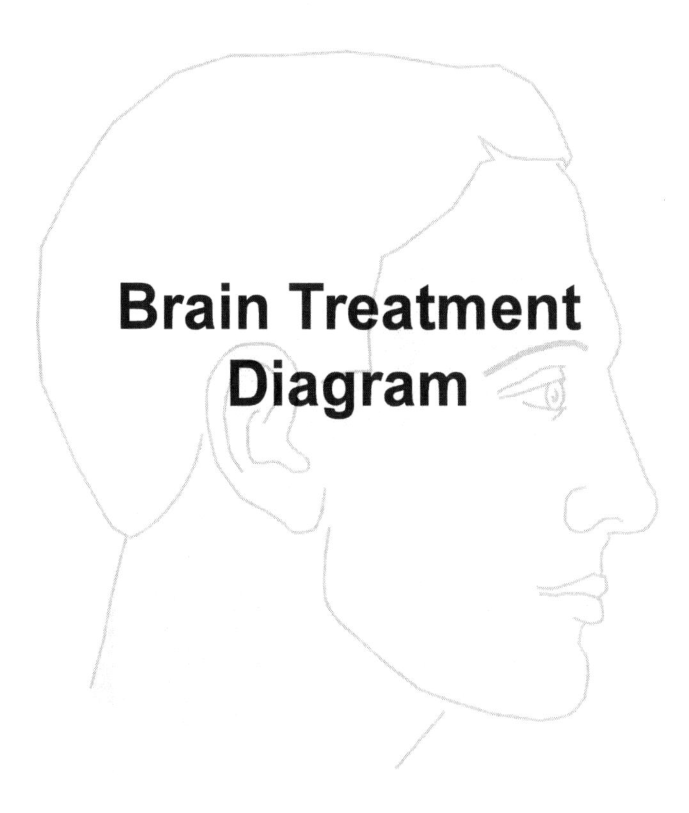
Brain Treatment
Diagram

Brain Treatment

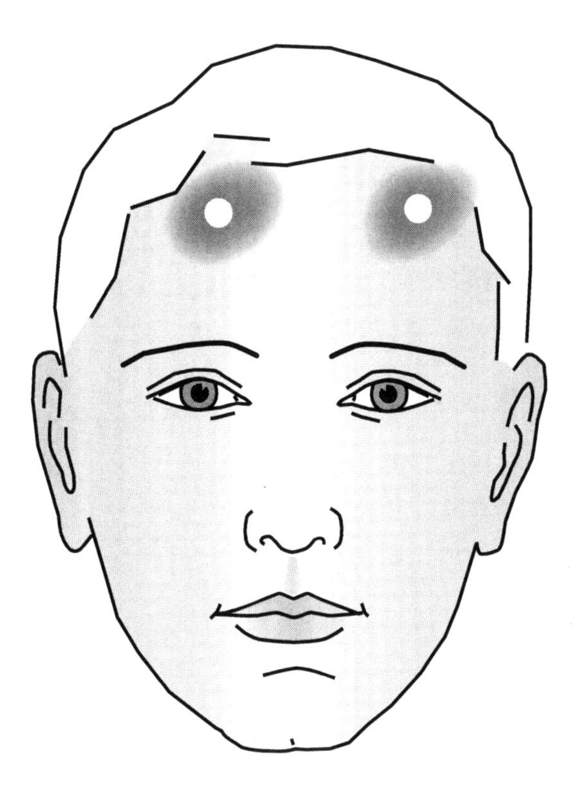

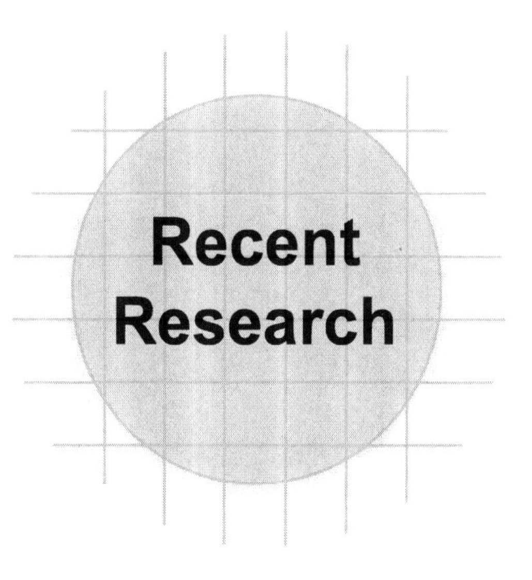
Recent
Research

AUTONOMIC NERVOUS SYSTEM BENEFITS
Irradiation of the Stellate Ganglion reduced VAS scores and increased local temp due to an increase regional blood flow by a reduction in vascular tone
Hashimoto et al., Laser Therapy 1997 (9) pp 7–12.

AUTONOMIC NERVOUS SYSTEM BENEFITS
LLLT improves ANS function
Lasers Surg Med. 2014 Dec;46(10):796–803.

BACTERIA AND VIRUSES
LLLT can inhibit some bacteria and viruses.
Lett Appl Microbiol. 2016 Mar;62(3):230–6.
Lasers Med Sci. 2016 Apr;31(3):549–56.
Antiviral Res. 2014 Oct;110:70-6.

BONE REGENERATION
Laser improves osteoblastic formation, bone strength in fractures, implant stability, and can improve osteonecrosis of the jaw.
Lasers Med Sci. 2010 Jul;25(4):559–69).
J Orthop Surg Res. 2010 Jan 4;5(1):1.
J Photochem Photobiol B. 2016 Oct;163:14–21.

CARDIAC PATHOLOGY BENEFITS
LLLT improves cardiac function.
Photomed Laser Surg. 2016 Nov;34(11):516–524
Lasers Med Sci. 2016 Nov 17.

CARPAL TUNNEL SYNDROME
Meta-analysis demonstrated that low-level laser improved hand grip, pain, and sensory nerve function.
Medicine (Baltimore).2016 Aug;95(31): 4424.

CELL AND PHYSIOLOGICAL BENEFITS

INCREASES: Cell proliferation, cell division, cell maturation, secretion of growth factors, wound healing, collagen production, wound strength, wound closer, fibroblasts, myofibroblasts, chondrocytes, epithelialization, skin circulation, oxygen supply, activity satellite cell cultures (stem cells).

DECREASES: Prostaglandin E2, substance P, cyclooxygenase 2 (Cox 2), muscle tension.

J Clin Las Med Surg 2004; 22 (2)141–150.

CELLULAR BENEFITS

INCREASES: Mitochondria and ATP production, Cytochrome oxidase and singlet oxygen, tissue regeneration genes and motor proteins, RNA DNA synthesis, growth factors, cell metabolism, angiogenesis, and mitosis.

Desmet K, et al. Photomed Laser Surg. 2006 Jun;24(2):121–128.

CORTISONE HAS SIMILAR EFFECTS AS LIGHT

Animal study; 810-nm laser was almost as good as cortisone at reducing swelling.

Higher doses showed most benefit.

Laser therapy reduced joint swelling and correlated with decreased serum prostaglandins.

Castano AP, Lasers Surg Med 2007 Jul;39(6):543–50.

CORTISONE IMPROVED WITH LLLT

Laser plus cortisone more effective than cortisone by itself.

Photomed Laser Surg. 2010 Oct;28(5):639–46.

DEPTH OF PENETRATION

LLLT passing through the skull with an 808 nm wavelength laser penetrated approximately 40 mm (1.6 inches).

Lasers Surg Med. 2015 Apr;47(4):312–22.

808 nm laser produced 1 mW/cm2 was achieved at 3.4 cm (1.36 inches), but for 980 nm achieved only 2.2 cm (less than 1 inch). It was determined that 808 nm of light penetrates as much as 54% deeper than 980 nm light.
Photomed Laser Surg. 2013 Apr;31(4):163–8.

FROZEN SHOULDER BENEFITS
A significant improvement in laser therapy compared to the control group.
The treatment group experienced significantly less pain and significantly improved disability scores. Range of motion in the treatment group was better than placebo.
Photomed Laser Surg. 2008 Mar 16.

HAIR LOSS
Meta-analysis of studies covered in this review found an overall improvement in hair regrowth, thickness, and patient satisfaction following LLLT.
Lasers Surg Med. 2016 Apr 25.

HIGHER DOSES INHIBIT
Lower Doses Stimulate, Higher Doses Inhibit. Using 14X the dose inhibited tissue repair.
J Biophotonics. 2016 Mar 15.

HIGHER DOSES INHIBIT
Lower Doses Stimulate, Higher Doses Inhibit
Cumulative effect of lower doses (2.5 or 5 J/cm(2)) determines the stimulatory effect, while multiple exposures at higher doses (16 J/cm(2)) result in an inhibitory effect with more damage.
Photomed Laser Surg. 2006 Dec;24(6):705–14.

INCREASE MOUTH OPENING, DECREASED MUSCULAR PAIN, DECREASED EATING DIFFICULTY, AND DECREASED TENDER POINTS

Photomed Laser Surg. 2006; 25 (5): 637–80.

INFLAMMATORY MEDIATOR INHIBITION

DECREASES: Inflammatory mediators, Cytokine receptors, Inflammatory proteins, Genes that code for inflammation, Proapoptotic proteins.

Desmet K, et al. Photomed Laser Surg. 2006 Jun;24(2):121–128.

INTENSITY OF THE LASER RADIATION WAS REDUCED BY 66% AFTER BEING TRANSMITTED THROUGH THE SKIN.

Most laser radiation was absorbed within the first 1mm of skin.

Acupunct Eletrother Res., 2007;321 (1–2);81-6.

LLLT BRAIN DISORDERS

Harvard research shows that LLLT is a promising treatment for many types of brain disorders.

BBA Clin. 2016 Oct 1;6:113–124.

LOWER POWER DENSITIES SHOWED BEST COLLAGEN STRUCTURE

The best organization of collagen were shown by the lower densities. All wavelengths and fluences used in this study were efficient at accelerating the healing process, with lower densities better than higher, hotter densities.

Photomed Laser Surg. 2006 Dec;24(6):754–8.

LLLT VS LOW-INTENSITY PULSED ULTRASOUND (LIPUS)

LIPUS enhanced bone repair by promoting bone resorption; LLLT accelerated this process through bone formation.

Photomed Laser Surg. 2006 Dec;24(6):735–40.

MEDICATION STRONGER WITH LIGHT
Laser Helps TB Treatment: Laser plus medication better than medication alone for tuberculosis.
Indian J Tuberc. 2010 Apr;57(2):80–6.

MITOCHONDRAL FUNCTION IMPROVED
Improves oxygen production, promoting cellular survival, Increased Cytochrome c oxidase—terminal enzyme of the electron transport chain and a strong photoacceptor and other mitochondral enzymes.
J Photochem Photobiol B. 2006 Nov 17.

MUSCLE PERFORMANCE AND LASER
Meta-analysis of 533 studies showed can increase in muscle mass after training, and a decrease in inflammation and oxidative stress in muscle biopsies.
J Biophotonics. 2016 Nov 22.

NECK PAIN BENEFITS
LLLT improves chronic neck pain and function.
Open Orthop J. 2013 Sep 20;7:396–419.

NERVE GROWTH STIMULATION
Controlled trial showed regeneration of sciatic nerve and myelination in rats.
Rochkind. Photomed & Laser Surg. 2007, 25(3): 137–143.

NERVE HEALING
LLLT accelerates peripheral nerve regeneration.
Lasers Med Sci. 2015 Dec;30(9):2319–24.

NON-STEROIDALS: COMPARATIVE EFFECT
LLLT reduces inflammation and improves function, in some cases superior to NSAIDs.

J Lasers Med Sci. 2016 Winter;7(1):45–50.

ORAL MUCOSITIS

LLLT reduces pain in chemotherapy induced oral mucositis.
J Lasers Med Sci. 2016 Winter;7(1):45–50.

PARKINSON'S IMPROVED WITH LIGHT

LLL improves nerve function with Parkinson's.
Molecular Degen 2009 Jun 17;4:26

PENETRATION UP TO 23 CM

Lasers and LED's of Optimal Wavelength Penetrate up to 23 cm (4 studies).
Desmet K, et al. Photomed Laser Surg. 2006 Jun;24(2):121–128.

PERIPHERAL NEUROPATHY

LLLT helps patients with diabetic peripheral neuropathy.
Acta Med Iran. 2013 Sep 9;51(8):543–7.

PHYSIOLOGICAL BENEFITS

INCREASES: cell proliferation, cell division, cell maturation, secretion of growth factors, wound healing, collagen production, wound strength, wound closer, fibroblasts, myofibroblasts, chondrocytes, epithelialization, skin circulation, oxygen supply, activity satellite cell cultures (stem cells).
DECREASES: Prostaglandin E2, substance P, cyclooxygenase 2 (Cox 2), muscle tension.
J Clin Las Med Surg 2004; 22 (2)141–150.

PSYCHIATRIC DISORDERS IMPROVED

LLL applied to skull decreased depression and anxiety.
Behavioral and Brain Functions, 2009, 5:46, 8 December 2009.

6% OF PHOTONS REACH SPINAL CORD

Applied directly to SP of porcine subjects; 6% of photons reached cord and increased CGRP/mRNA.
Kimberly Byrnes, PhD, NAALT, 2003/2004.

STROKE

Animal Study; Neurological deficits improved.
Lasers Surg Med. 2006 Jan;38(1):70–3.
Stroke. 2006 Oct;37(10):2620–4.

STROKE HELPED WITH LIGHT

Laser applied to skull improves brain following stroke.
Curr Cardiol Rep. 2010 Jan;12(1):29–33

TEMPORMANDIBULAR JOINT (TMJ)

Decrease of pain and anti-inflammatory effects; confirmed by thermographic examination.
Photomed Laser Surg. 2006 Aug;24(4):522–7.

TENDINITIS AND MYOFASCIAL PAIN BENEFITS

Acute tendinitis had the best response.
Logdberg-Anersson et al., Laser Therapy 1997 (9) pp 79–86.

TENDINITIS BENEFITS

LLLT proven to help tendinitis.
Acta Ortop Bras. 2015 Jan-Feb;23(1):47–9.

THYROID FUNCTION IMPROVES

Laser improves the function of the thyroid based on lab values with chronic autoimmune thyroiditis.
Lasers Surg Med. 2010 Aug;42(6):589–96.

Bibliography

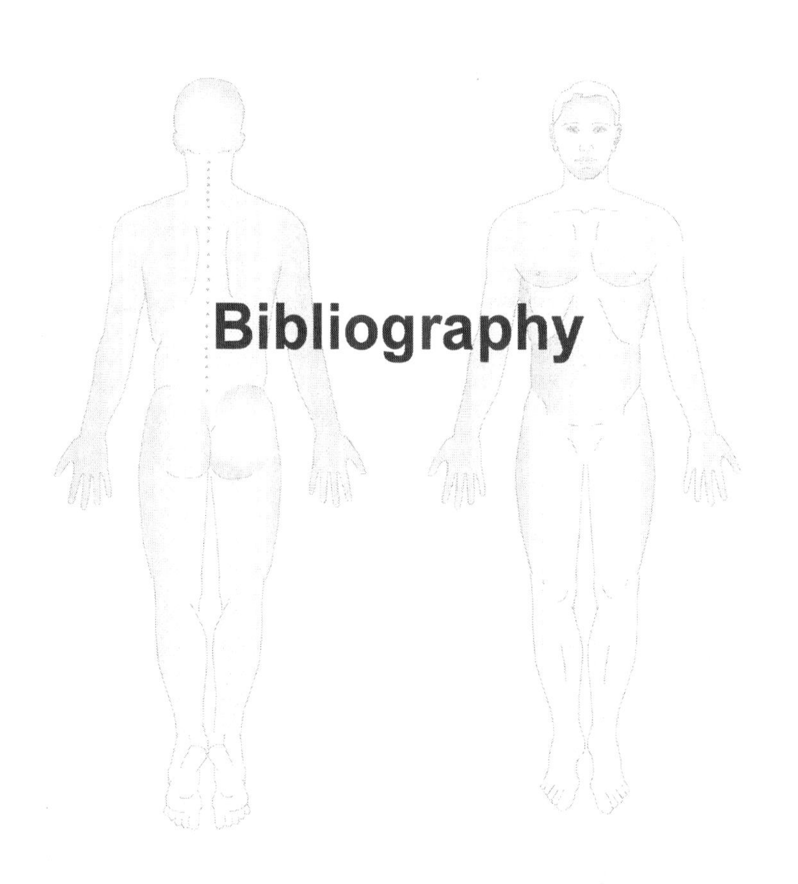

Ad N and Oron U. (2001): Impact of low energy laser irradiation on infarct size in the rat following myocardial infarction. Inter. J. Cardiol, 80:109–116.

Aimbire F, Albertini R, de Magalhães R G, Lopes-Martins R A et al. Effect of LLLT Ga-Al-As (685 nm) on LPS-induced inflammation of the airway and lung in the rat. Lasers in Medical Science. 2005; 20 (1): 11–20.

Aimbire F, Albertini R, Leonardo P, Castro Faria Neto HC, Iversen V V, Lopes-Martins R A B, Bjordal J M. Low level laser therapy induces dose-dependent reduction of TNF-alpha levels in acute inflammation. Photomed Laser Surg. 2006; 24 (1): 33–37.

Al-Watban F A, Zhang X Y. The comparison of effects between pulsed and CW lasers on wound healing. J Clin Laser Med Surg. 2004; 22 (1):15–18.

Amat A, Rigau J, Nicolau R, Aalders M et al. Effect of red and near-infrared laser light on adenosine triphosphate (ATP) in the luciferine-luciferase reaction. Journal of Photochemistry and Photobiology A: Chemistry. 2004; 168 (1–2): 59–65.

Anders J J, Geuna S, Rochkind S. Phototherapy promotes regeneration and functional recovery of injured peripheral nerve. Neurol Res. 2004; 26 (2): 233–239.

Bagis S, Comelekoglu U, Coskun B, Milcan A et al. No effect of GA-AS (904 nm) laser irradiation on the intact skin of the injured rat sciatic nerve. Lasers in Medical Science. 2003; 18 (2): 83–88.

Bakhtiary A H, Rashidy-Pour A. Ultrasound and laser therapy in the treatment of carpal tunnel syndrome. Aust J Physiother. 2004; 50: 147–151.

Bayat M, Delbari A, Almaseyeh M A et al. Low-level laser therapy improves early healing of medial collateral ligament injuries in rats. Photomed Laser Surg. 2005; 23 (6): 556–560.

Bayat M, Vasheghani M M, Razavi N et al. Effect of low-level laser therapy on the healing of second-degree burns in rats: a histological and microbiological study. J Photochem Photobiol B. 2005; 78 (2): 171–177.

Berman, MH. Photobiomodulation with Near Infrared Light Helmet in a Pilot, Placebo Controlled Clinical Trial in Dementia Patients Testing Memory and Cognition J Neurol Neurosci. 2017; 8(1).

Bjordal J M, Johnson M I, Iversen V, Aimbire F, Lopes-Martins R A. Photoradiation in acute pain: a systematic review of possible mechanisms of action and clinical effects in randomized placebo-controlled trials. Photomed Laser Surg. 2006; 24 (2): 158–168.

Bjordal J M, Lopes-Martins R A, Iversen V V. A randomised, placebo controlled trial of low level laser therapy for activated Achilles tendinitis with microdialysis measurement of peritendinous prostaglandin E2 concentrations. Br J Sports Med. 2006; 40 (1): 76–80.

Bjordal J M. Can a Cochrane review in controversial areas be biased? A sensitivity analysis based on the protocol of a systematic Cochrane review Low Level Laser Therapy in Osteoarthritis. Photomed Laser Surg. 2005; 23 (5): 453–458.

Byrnes K R, Barna L, Chenault V M et al. Photobiomodulation improves cutaneous wound healing in an animal model of type II diabetes. Photomed Laser Surg. 2004; 22 (4): 281–290.

Byrnes K R, Waynant R W, Ilev I K Wu X et al. Light promotes regeneration and functional recovery and alters the immune response after spinal cord injury. Lasers Surg Med. 2005; 36 (3): 171–185.

Byrnes K R, Wu X, Waynant R W, Ilev I K, Anders J J. Low power laser irradiation alters gene expression of olfactory ensheathing cells in vitro. Lasers Surg Med. 2005; 37 (2): 161–117.

Chow R T, Barnsley L. Systematic review of the literature of low-level laser therapy (LLLT) in the management of neck pain. Lasers Surg Med. 2005; 37 (1): 46–52.

Chow RT, Heller GZ, Barnsley L. The effect of 300mW, 830nm laser on chronic neck pain: A double-blind, randomized, placebo-controlled study. Pain. 2006 Sep;124(1-2):201–10.

Crespi R, Covani U, Margarone JE, Andreana S. (1997): Periodontal tissue regeneration in beagle dogs after laser therapy. Lasers Surg Med, 21:395–402.

Croghan IT, et al. A randomized, open-label pilot of the combination of low-level laser therapy and lorcaserin for weight loss. 2016: BMC Obes. Sep 29;3:42.

de Medeiros JS, Vieira GF, Nishimura PY. Laser application effects on the bite strength of the masseter muscle, as an orofacial pain treatment. Photomed Laser Surg. 2005; 23 (4): 373–376.

Devor M. (1990): What's in a beam for pain therapy? Pain, 43:139.

Dyson M, and Young S. (1986): Effect of laser therapy on wound contraction and cellularity in mice. Lasers in Medical Science, 1:125–130.

Ebneshahidi N S, Heshmatipour M, Moghaddami A, Eghtesadi A P. The effects of laser acupuncture on chronic tension headache—a randomised controlled trial. Acupuncture in Medicine. 2005; 23 (1): 13-18.

Fargas-Babjak A. (2001): Acupuncture, transcutaneous electrical nerve stimulation, and laser therapy in chronic pain. Clin J Pain, 17(4 Suppl):S105–13.

Fillipin L I, Mauriz J L, Vedovelli K, Moreira A J, Zettler C G, Lech O, Marroni N P, Gonzalez-Gallego J. Low-level laser therapy (LLLT) prevents oxidative stress and reduces fibrosis in rat traumatized Achilles tendon. Lasers Surg Med. 2005; 37 (4): 293–300.

Gigo-Benato D, Geuna S, de Castro Rodrigues A, Tos P et al. Low-power laser bio-stimulation enhances nerve repair after end-to-side neurorrhaphy: a double-blind randomized study in the rat median nerve model. Lasers in Medical Science, 2004; 19 (1): 57–65.

Gottlieb T, Jörgensen B, Rohde E, Müller G, Schellera EE. The influence of irradiation with low-level diode laser on the proteoglycan content in arthrotically changed cartilage in rabbits. Medical Laser Application. 2006; 21 (1): 53–59.

Gruber W, Eber E, Malle-Scheid D, Pfleger A et al. Laser acupuncture in children and adolescents with exercise induced asthma. Thorax. 2002; 57 (3): 222–225.

Gür A, Cosut A, Sarac A J et al. Effect of different therapy regimes of low power laser in painful osteoarthritis of the knee: A double-blind and placebo-controlled trial. Lasers in Surgery and Medicine. 2003; 33: 330–338.

Gür A, Karakoc M, Cevik R et al. Efficacy of low power laser therapy and exercise on pain and functions in chronic low back pain. Lasers in Surgery and Medicine. 2003; 32 (3): 233–238.

Gür A, Sarac A J, Cevik R, Altindag O, Sarac S. Efficacy of 904 nm gallium arsenide low level laser therapy in the management of chronic myofascial pain in the neck: a double-blind and randomized-controlled trial. Lasers in Surgery and

Medicine. 2004; 35 (3):229–235.

Gür A,Cosut A, Sarac A et al. Efficacy of different therapy regimes of low-power laser in painful osteoarthritis of the knee: a double-blind and randomized-controlled trial. Laser Surg Med. 2003; 33: 330–338.

Hawkins DH, Abrahamse H. The role of laser fluence in cell viability, proliferation, and membrane integrity of wounded human skin fibroblasts following helium-neon laser irradiation. Lasers Surg Med. 2006; 38 (1): 74–83.

Ihsan F R. Low-level laser therapy accelerates collateral circulation and enhances microcirculation. Photomed Laser Surg. 2005; 23 (3): 289–294.

Iijima K, Shimoyama N, Shimoyama M, Yamamoto T, Shimizu T, and Mizuguchi T (1989): Effect of repeated irradiation of low-power He-Ne laser in pain relief from postherpetic neuralgia. Clin J Pain, 5: 271–274.

Karu, T. Photobiology of low-power laser effects. Health Physics, 1989: 56, 691-704.

Khadra M, Kassem N, Haanaes H R, Ellingsen J E, Lyngstadaas S P. Enhancement of bone formation in rat calvarial bone defects using low-level laser therapy. Oral Surg Oral Med Oral Pathol Oral Endod. 2004; 97: 693–700.

Laakso E L, Cabot P J. Nociceptive scores and endorphin-containing cells reduced by low-level laser therapy (LLLT) in inflamed paws of Wistar rat. Photomed Laser Surg. 2005; 23 (1): 32–35.

Lanzafame R J, Stadler I, Coleman J, Haerum B, Oskoui P, Whittaker M, Zhang R Y. Temperature-controlled 830-nm low-level laser therapy of experimental pressure ulcers. Photomed Laser Surg. 2004; 22 (6): 483–488.

Lopes-Martins R A, Albertini R, Martins P S, Bjordal J M, Faria Neto H C. Spontane-ous effects of low-level laser therapy (650 nm) in acute inflammatory mouse pleurisy induced by carrageenan. Photomed Laser Surg. 2005; 23 (4): 377–381.

Lopes-Martins R A, Marcos R L, Leonardo P S, Prianti A C, Muscara M, Aimbire F N, Frigo L, Iversen V V, Bjordal J M. The Effect of Low Level Laser Irradiation (Ga-Al-As - 655nm) On Skeletal Muscle Fatigue induced by Electrical Stimulation in Rats. J Appl Physiol. 2006 Apr 20.

Mendez T M, Pinheiro A L, Pacheco M T, Nascimento P M, Ramalho L M. Dose and wavelength of laser light have influence on the repair of cutaneous wounds. J Clin Laser Med Surg. 2004; 22 (1): 19–25.

Mognato M, Squizzato F, Facchin F, Zaghetto L, Corti L. Cell growth modulation of human cells irradiated in vitro with low-level laser therapy. Photomed Laser Surg. 2004; 22 (6): 523–526.

Monteforte P, Baratto L, Molfetta L, Rovetta G. Low-power laser in osteoarthritis of the cervical spine. Int J Tissue React. 2003; 25 (4):131–136.

Naeser M, Hahn K-A, Lieberman BE, Branco KF. (2002): Carpal Tunnel Syndrome Pain Treated with Low-Level Laser and Microamperes Transcutaneous Electric Nerve Stimulation: A Controlled Study. Archives of Physical Medicine and Rehabilitation, 83:978–988.

Nakaji S, Shiroto C, Yodono M, Umeda T, Liu Q. Retrospective study of adjunctive diode laser therapy for pain attenuation in 662 patients: detailed analysis by questionnaire. Photomed Laser Surg. 2005; 23 (1): 60–65.

Nascimento P M, Pinheiro A L, Salgado M A, Ramalho L M. A preliminary report on the effect of laser therapy on the healing of cutaneous surgical wounds as a consequence of an inversely proportional relationship between wavelength and intensity: histological study in rats. Photomed Laser Surg. 2004; 22 (6):513–518.

Nicola R A, Jorgetti V, Rigau J, Marcos T T. Effect of low-power GaAlAs laser (660 nm) on bone structure and cell activity: an experimental animal study. Lasers in Medical Science 2003; 18 (2): 89–94.

Oren DA, Charney DS, Lavie R, Sinyakov M, Lubart R. (2001): Stimulation of reactive oxygen species production by an antidepressant visible light source. Biol Psychiatry, 49:464–467.

Oron U, Yaakobi T, Oron A, Hayam G, Gepstein L, Wolf T and Ben Haim S. (2001): Attenuation of the formation of scar tissue in rats and dogs post myocardial infarction by low energy laser irradiation. Lasers Surg. Med, 28:204–211.

Oron U, Yaakobi T, Oron A, Mordechovitz D, Shofti R, Hayam G, Dror U, Gepstein L, Wolf T, Haudenschild C and Ben Haim S. (2001): Low energy laser irradiation reduces formation of scar tissue following myocardial infarction in dogs. Circulation, 93:296–301.

Oron U. Photoengineering of tissue repair in skeletal and cardiac muscles. Photomed Laser surg. 2006; 24 (2): 111–120.

Ozkan N, Altan L, Bingol U et al. Investigation of the supplementary effect of GaAs laser therapy on the rehabilitation of human digital flexor tendons. J Clin Laser Med Surg. 2004; 22 (2):105–110.

Ozdemir F, Birtane M, Kokino S. (2001): The clinical efficacy of low-power laser therapy on pain and function in cervical osteoarthritis. Clin Rheumatol, 20(3):181–4.

Pinfildi C E, Liebano R E, Hochman B S, Ferreira L M. Helium-neon laser in viability of random skin flap in rats. Lasers Surg Med. 2005; 37 (1): 74–77.

Reddy GK, Stehno-Bittel L, Enwemeka CS. (2001): Laser photostimulation accelerates wound healing in diabetic rats. Wound Repair and Regeneration, 9.

Salate A C, Barbosa G, Gaspar P et al. Effect of Ga-Al-As Diode Laser Irradiation on Angiogenesis in Partial Ruptures of Achilles Tendon in Rats. Photomed Laser Surg. 2005; 23 (5): 470–475.

Schiling L, et al. 1060 nm Diode Hyperthermic Laser Lipolysis: The Latest in Non-Invasive Body Contouring. J Drugs Dermatol. 2017: Jan 1;16(1):48-52.

Siedentopf C M, , Koppelstaetter F, Haala I A et al. Laser acupuncture induced specific cerebral cortical and subcortical activations in humans. Lasers in Medical Science. 2005; July 1.

Smith, KC. Photomed Laser Surg. 2005: Feb;23(1):78-80.

Soriano F, Campaña V, Moya M, Gavotto A et al. Photobiomodulation of pain and inflammation on microcrystalline arthropathies: experimental and clinical results. Photomed Laser Surg. 2006; 24 (2): 140–150.

Tunér J and Hode L. (2002): Laser Therapy—Clinical Practice and Scientific Background. Sweden. Prima Books.

Whelan, H.T. et al. Effect of NASA Light-Emitting Diode Irradiationon Wound Healing. Journal of Clinical Laser Medicine & Surgery. 2001: 19 (6). 2.

Wong B J, Pandhoh N, Truong M T, Diaz S et al. Identification of chondrocyte proliferation following laser irradiation, thermal injury, and mechanical trauma. Lasers Surg Med. 2005; 37 (1): 89–96.

Yasuyo M, Toshiyuki I, Toyoshi H, Kazuhiro Y, and Mayumi N. (2000): Effects of Near-Infrared Low Level Laser irradiation on microcirculation. Lasers Surg Med, 27:427–437.

Glossary

Absorb: To transform radiant energy into a different form, with a resultant rise in temperature.

Absorption: Transformation of radiant energy to a different form of energy by the interaction of matter, depending on temperature and wavelength.

Absorption Coefficient: Factor describing light's ability to be absorbed per unit of path length.

Active Medium: Collection of atoms or molecules capable of undergoing stimulated emission at a given wavelength.

Amplitude: The maximum value of the electromagnetic wave, measured from the mean to the extreme; simply stated: the height of the wave.

Aperture: An opening through which radiation can pass.

Attenuation: The decrease in energy (or power) as a beam passes through an absorbing or scattering medium.

Average Power: The total energy imparted during exposure divided by the exposure duration.

Beam: A collection of rays that may be parallel, convergent, or divergent.

Brightness: The visual sensation of the luminous intensity of a light source. The brightness of a laser beam is most closely associated with the radiometric concept of radiance.

Cathode: A negatively charged electrical element providing electrons for an electrical discharge.

Convergence: The bending of light rays toward each other, as by a positive (convex) lens.

Dosimetry: Measurement of the power, energy, irradiance, or radiant exposure of light delivered to tissue.

Electromagnetic Radiation: The propagation of varying electric and magnetic fields through space at the velocity of light.

Electromagnetic Spectrum: The range of frequencies and wavelengths emitted by atomic systems. The total spectrum includes radio waves as well as short cosmic rays.

Electromagnetic Wave: A disturbance which propagates outward from an electric charge that oscillates or is accelerated. Includes radio waves; x-rays; gamma rays; and infrared, ultraviolet, and visible light.

Electron: Negatively charged particle of an atom.

Emission: Act of giving off radiant energy by an atom or molecule.

Emissivity: The ratio of the radiant energy emitted by any source to that emitted by a blackbody at the same temperature.

Energy: The product of power (watts) and duration (seconds). One watt second = one joule.

Flux: The radiant, or luminous, power of a light beam; the time rate of the flow of radiant energy across a given surface.

Focal Length: Distance between the center of a lens and the point on the optical axis to which parallel rays of light are converged by the laser.

Focus: As a noun, the point where rays of light meet which

have been reflected by a mirror or refracted by a lens, giving rise to an image of the source. As a verb, to adjust focal length for the clearest image and smallest spot size.

Frequency: The number of light waves passing a fixed point in a given unit of time, or the number of complete vibrations in that period of time.

Gaussian Curve: Statistical curve showing a peak with normal even distribution on either side. May either be a sharp peak with steep sides, or a blunt peak with shallower sides. Used to show power distribution in a beam. The concept is important in controlling the geometry of the light's impact.

Ground State: Lowest energy level of an atom.

Incident Light: A ray of light that falls on the surface of a lens or any other object. The "angle of incidence" is the angle made by the ray with a perpendicular (normal) to the surface.

Infrared Radiation (IR): Invisible electromagnetic radiation with wavelengths which lie within the range of 0.70 to 1000 micrometers.

Intensity: The magnitude of radiant energy.

Ionizing Radiation: Radiation commonly associated with x-ray or other high energy electromagnetic radiation which will cause DNA damage with no direct, immediate thermal effect. Contrasts with non-ionizing radiation of lasers.

Irradiance (E): Radiant flux (radiant power) per unit area incident upon a given surface. Units: Watts per square centimeter. (Sometimes referred to as power density.)

Irradiation: Exposure to radiant energy, such as heat, x-rays, or light.

Joule (J): A unit of energy (1 watt-second) used to describe the rate of energy delivery.

Joule/cm2: A unit of radiant exposure used in measuring the amount of energy incident upon a unit area.

Laser: An acronym for light amplification by stimulated emission of radiation. A laser is a cavity, with mirrors at the ends, filled with material such as crystal, glass, liquid, gas, or dye.

Lens: A curved piece of optically transparent material which depending on its shape is used to either converge or diverge light.

Light: The range of electromagnetic radiation frequencies detected by the eye, or the wavelength range from about 400 to 760 nanometers.

Monochromatic Light: Theoretically, light consisting of just one wavelength. No light is absolutely single frequency since it will have some bandwidth. Lasers provide the narrowest of bandwidths that can be achieved.

Nanometer (nm): A unit of length in the International System of Units (SI) equal to one billionth of a meter. Abbreviated nm—a measure of length. One nm equals 10^{-9} meter, and is the usual measure of light wavelengths. Visible light ranges from about 400 nm in the purple to about 760 nm in the deep red.

Optical Radiation: Ultraviolet, visible, and infrared radiation (0.35–1.4 nm) that falls in the region of transmittance of the human eye.

Output Power: The energy per second measured in watts emitted from the light device.

Phase: Waves are in phase with each other when all the troughs and peaks coincide and are "locked" together. The result is a reinforced wave in increased amplitude (brightness).

Photon: In quantum theory, the elemental unit of light, having both wave and particle behavior. It has motion, but no mass or charge.

Power: The rate of energy delivery expressed in watts (joules per second). Thus: 1 Watt = 1 joule/1 Sec.

Radiance Brightness: The radiant power per unit solid angle and per unit area of a radiating surface.

Radiation: In the context of optics, electromagnetic energy is released; the process of releasing electromagnetic energy.

Reflection: The return of radiant energy (incident light) by a surface, with no change in wavelength.

Refraction: The change of direction of propagation of any wave, such as an electromagnetic wave, when it passes from one medium to another in which the wave velocity is different. The bending of incident rays as they pass from one medium to another (e.g., air to glass).

Ruby: The first laser type; a crystal of sapphire (aluminum oxide) containing trace amounts of chromium oxide.

Spot Size: The mathematical measurement of the radius of the light beam.

Transmission: Passage of electromagnetic radiation through a medium.

Visible Radiation (light): Electromagnetic radiation which can be detected by the human eye. It is commonly used to describe wavelengths which lie in the range between 400 nm and 700–780 nm. The peak of the human spectral response is about 555 nm.

Watt: A unit of power (equivalent to one joule per second) used to express laser power.

Watt/cm2: A unit of irradiance used in measuring the amount of power per area of absorbing surface, or per area of the light beam.

Wave: A sinusoidal undulation or vibration; a form of movement by which all radiant electromagnetic energy travels.

Wavelength: The length of the light wave, usually measured from peak to peak, which determines its color. The common unit of measurement is the nanometer.

Index

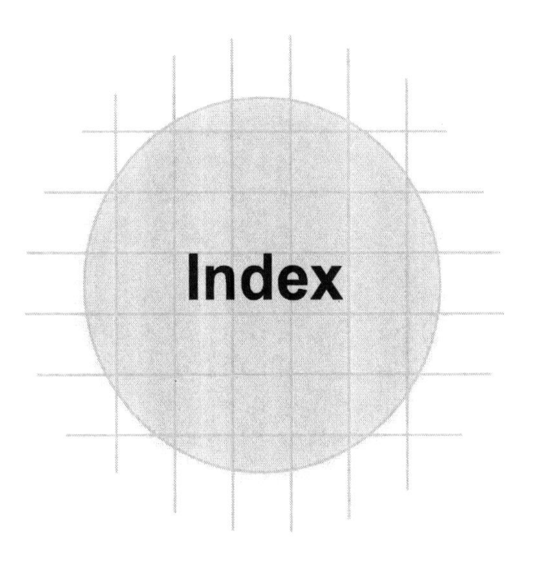